Romeo et Rock

MW01119836

ALICE STREET

Footprints Series
JANE ERRINGTON, Editor

The life stories of individual women and men who were participants in interesting events help nuance larger historical narratives, at times reinforcing those narratives, at other times contradicting them. The Footprints series introduces extraordinary Canadians, past and present, who have led fascinating and important lives at home and throughout the world.

The series includes primarily original manuscripts but may consider the English-language translation of works that have already appeared in another language. The editor of the series welcomes inquiries from authors. If you are in the process of completing a manuscript that you think might fit into the series, please contact her, care of McGill-Queen's University Press, 3430 McTavish Street, Montreal, QC H3A 1X9.

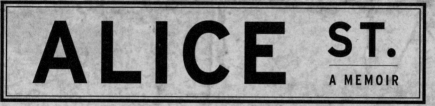

ALICE ST.

A MEMOIR

RICHARD VALERIOTE

McGILL-QUEEN'S UNIVERSITY PRESS

Montreal & Kingston · London · Ithaca

© McGill-Queen's University Press 2010

ISBN 978-0-7735-3654-8

Legal deposit first quarter 2010
Bibliothèque nationale du Québec

Printed in Canada on acid-free paper that is 100% ancient forest free
(100% post-consumer recycled), processed chlorine free.

McGill-Queen's University Press acknowledges the support of the Canada Council for
the Arts for our publishing program. We also acknowledge the financial support of the
Government of Canada through the Book Publishing Industry Development Program
(BPIDP) for our publishing activities.

Library and Archives Canada Cataloguing in Publication

Valeriote, Richard, 1929–
Alice Street : A Memoir / Richard Valeriote.
(Footprints series ; no. 12)
ISBN 978-0-7735-3654-8
1. Valeriote, Richard M., 1929–. 2. Italian Canadians--Biography.
3. Physicians–Canada–Biography.
I. Title. II. Series: Footprints series no. 12

R464.V34A3 2010   610.69'5092   C2009-904666-0

This book was designed and typeset by studio oneonone in Sabon 10.2/14.2

To my lifelong partner,

Polly,

without whose help none of this

would have been possible.

CONTENTS

FAMILY ALBUM

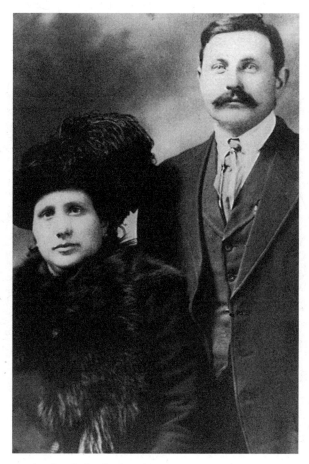

Michael and Elizabeth Valeriote, 1920

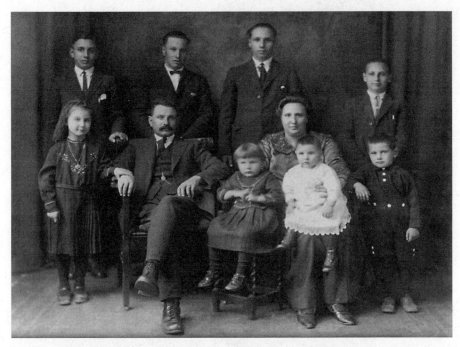

The first half of the family in 1923: back row left to right – Silvio, Dominic, Michael, Steve; front row left to right – Mary, Father (Michael Sr), Mother (Elizabeth) holding Savina and Palma, Pacifico

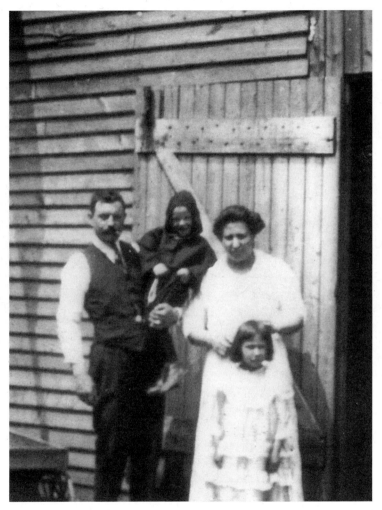

Father, Pacifico in his Saint Anthony outfit, Mother, and my sister Mary.

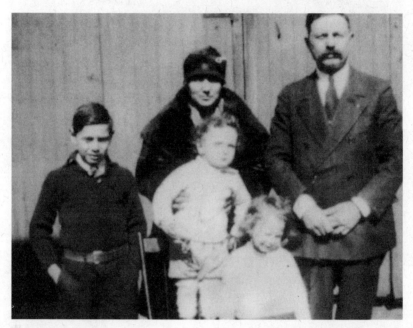

The Valeriotes ca 1920. Left to right, Pacifico, Mother, holding Richard and Gertrude, Father

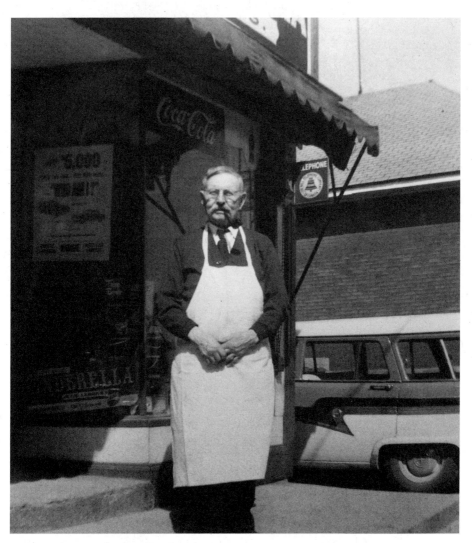

My father in front of the store, 1940

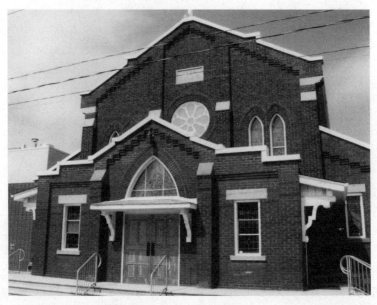

Sacred Heart Church, 1950

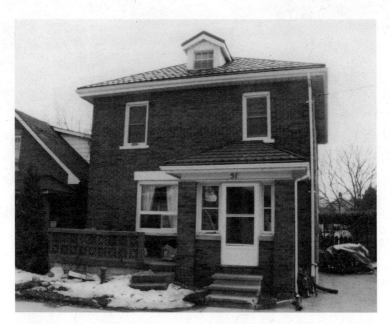

Our house on Alice Street, 1954

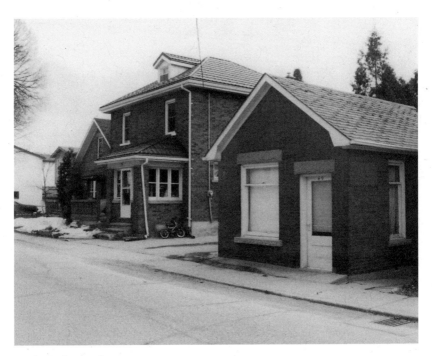

Uncle Vincent's shop, 1950

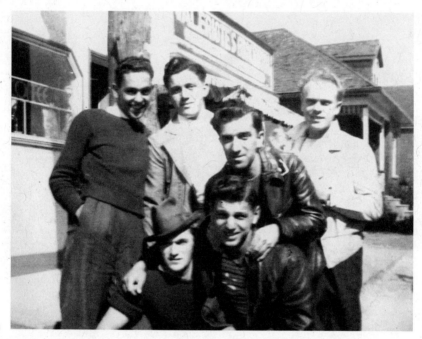

Some of the young men in the neighborhood: back row, left to right, Cosmo Ferraro, Ralph Sorbara, Mitch Doibyk, Odo Melason; front row, left to right, Mike Worunka, Jimmy Valeriote

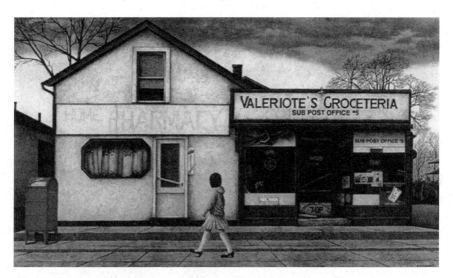

The Family Store where I worked for nine years and three months, as shown in "Sunday Morning" by G.W. Campbell (28″ × 24″, egg tempera on panel, completed 1998).

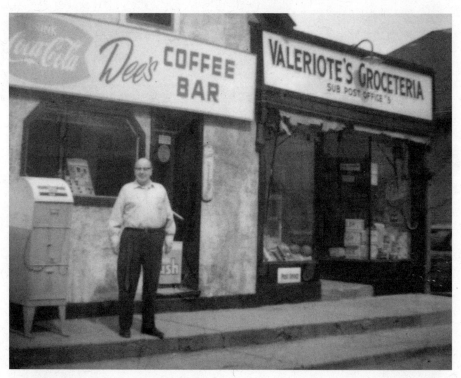

My brother Dominic next to the store, 1950

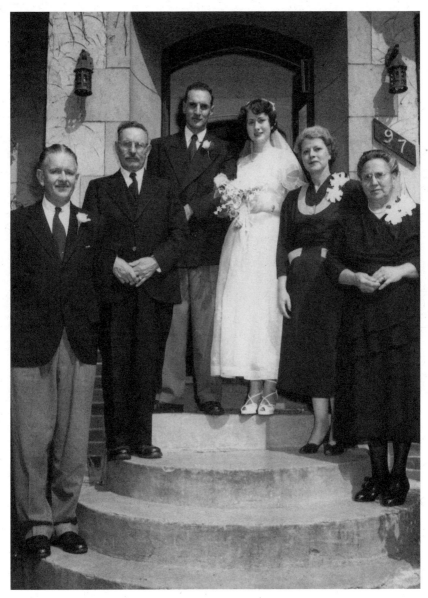

Our wedding, St Brigid's Church in Ottawa, 1951. Standing with us are our parents, Frederick and Pauline Pillet and Michael and Elizabeth Valeriote.

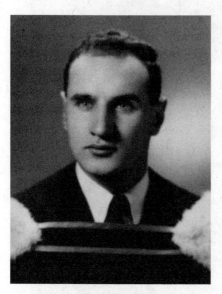

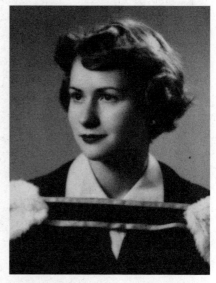

My graduation picture, McGill 1952   Polly's graduation picture, McGill 1953

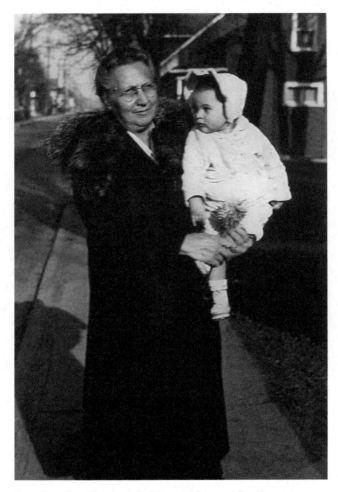

Grandmother Elizabeth holding Cathy on Alice Street, 1954

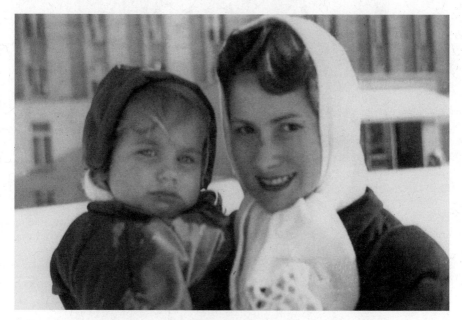

Polly with Susie, in front of St. Joseph's Hospital, 1955

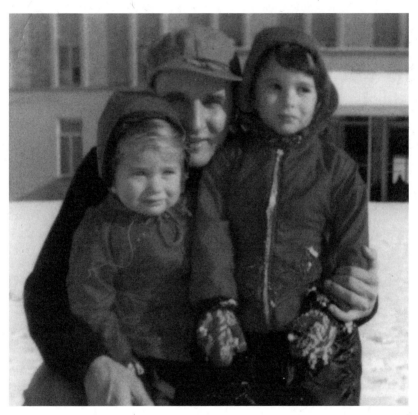

Richard with Susie and Cathy, in front of St. Joseph's Hospital, 1955

PART I

THE WARD

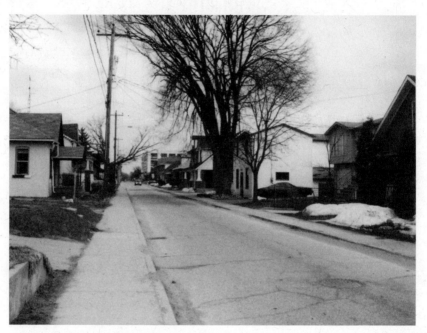

Looking down Alice Street

CHAPTER ONE
BORN AT THE DAWN OF HARD TIMES

The long, improbable journey that delivered me to the lecture halls and dissection labs at McGill University Medical School on my way to a doctor's life began in the immigrant neighborhood of Alice Street in Guelph, Ontario. It was improbable because I had to grow up fast, flirted with the Grim Reaper once or twice, went to bed hungry more nights than I care to remember, and survived thanks to a series of small miracles facilitated by family, friends, and strangers alike. If I hadn't lived it, I'd swear it was fiction.

It seems fitting now that my life began just a couple of months before the Wall Street Crash of October 1929 that killed off the Roaring Twenties and ushered in the Great Depression. Born 5 August, I was my mother's fifteenth child and her next to last. I arrived at the sunset of the good times – my father was at the peak of his prosperity – and the dawn of hard ones. Adversity had plenty of company in "The Ward," as the neighborhood was known – short for St Patrick's Ward. Our house was on Alice Street, a half-mile stretch of modest homes that was a distinct community to those who lived on it. It was an ethnically rich, culturally proud neighborhood of working-class strivers in Guelph's industrial zone.

Several rail lines, spurs, and factory sidings converged at a locomotive roundhouse where a shuttle engine was parked at night and fired up in the morning to move box and tanker cars to and from the pipe, rubber, and appliance plants.

On a hot summer evening, with windows thrown open and people sitting on their stoops to escape the heat, the short walk from one end of Alice Street to the other exposed you to the full spectrum of Europe's mother tongues and accents: Irish, Scottish, British, French, German, Polish, Russian, Spanish.

The predominant language was Italian, the language I grew up hearing and speaking at home. Many of the Italians in Guelph had emigrated as family groups from the southern Italian hill town of San Giorgio Morgeto, which sits atop a steep-sided hill at the edge of the Aspromonte ("Sour Mountains") region, so named by local farmers because of its steep terrain and rocky soil. A cluster of densely packed, tile-roofed buildings separated by narrow, cobble-stoned streets and dominated by a castle nestled among forested foothills, today it would be regarded as a charming ochre-walled vacation stop in sunny Italy. In 1900, its 4,000 or so residents saw it as a hardscrabble backwater in the impoverished region of Calabria, a pebble in the toe of Italy's boot. At the turn of the century, when my father was a young man eager to make his mark on the world, there was no charm in the bleak future offered by San Giorgio.

One of the first members of my family to arrive in North America was Salvatore Valeriote (in some records the name is spelled Valerioti). Salvatore is listed in the records at Ellis Island, New York, as a thirty-seven-year-old married farmer who arrived by ship on 26 April 1903. Several dozen other men from San Giorgio arrived on the same boat, destined for Montreal where they had been promised jobs working on the railroads.

My parents, Michele (Michael) and Elisabetta (Elizabeth), arrived in Guelph during those early years of the century. My father had preceded my mother and lived in a dormitory with other immigrants until he saved enough from work in the local pipe factory to return to San Giorgio to fetch her. Their first child, my eldest brother, Dominic, was born in Guelph in 1906.

By the time I arrived, I had brothers old enough to be my father, and my father was old enough to be my grandfather. At family occasions such as weddings and Christmas, the entire Valeriote family seemed to descend upon us, swelling our ranks to two dozen or so. For years I was confused about who all these adults were, chattering away in Italian and greeting each other with old world rituals.

My father had become a successful merchant. He owned the local grocery store, served as the local post master, and was the landlord of several small apartment houses.

Although my parents brought a lot of children into the world, all of us were never in the same place at the same time. Dominic was twenty-five years old with a family of his own when Anna, my younger sister and my mother's last child, was born in 1931.

By 1929, when I was born, six of our siblings had died in childhood and four – Dominic and the three brothers born after him – had left home. There were six of us children in the house, including the oldest girls, Mary and Savina, both of whom soon after got married and moved out. Later, when World War II broke out, my older brother Pacifico left for military duty, reducing our ranks to three: two sisters and myself. We picked up one when a niece whose mother came down with tuberculosis spent a couple of years in our home.

My father was a passionate and generous man whose good nature and kind heart proved his undoing when the Depression took hold and his customers began to come up short in food money. He extended credit until many of those folks got so far behind they quit coming around. He refused to pursue them, convinced God would frown on his suing the poor.

He also couldn't say no to his children. When two of my brothers, Mike and Silvio, were accepted to attend the University of Western Ontario, Pa sold one of his apartment buildings to raise the money for tuition. He'd spent $12,000 to build it in the 1920s, but in the depths of the Depression it fetched just $2,000. Not only did he lose $10,000, but he sacrificed the income the building had been generating.

Both Mike and Silvio put the money to good use, graduating and going on to productive careers. (Mike became a teacher and Silvio a physician, inspiring my interest in medicine.) But my father's financial fortunes and self-esteem never recovered. Adding to his woes was a ruptured appendix in 1931 that nearly killed him.

As his fortunes and health sagged, he slipped into depression. He became so incapacitated that Dominic decided to come home and see what he could do. He'd been living in Detroit where, as a young man with an eighth-grade education, he'd gone to seek a future. He had married and settled there, working in a Ford Motor Company plant.

My father's business was in such a sad state that when Dominic insisted that he should take it over and be the boss, my father was in no position to debate. In the process of assessing the situation, Dominic discovered in a cabinet several tattered macaroni boxes stuffed with old, unpaid grocery bills, rolled up in bundles held together by rubber bands – thousands of dollars of worthless paper.

Dominic returned to Guelph with not only his wife but an entourage of in-laws: his wife's elderly father and two brothers with their wives. Three of the in-laws went to work in the store and in an adjacent coffee bar. Dominic also took over our living quarters behind the store. My parents and siblings and I moved down the street, to the house where I lived off and on until I was twenty-eight. Pa continued to work in the store, but ever after answered to Dominic.

My father seemed to become an old man overnight. He remained depressed the rest of his life and I scarcely remember him speaking more than a few words now and then in the years I lived at home. We did, however, find a way to connect. He'd sit for hours by the radio, smoking his pipe, listening to opera, and deciphering as best he could the news in the English language paper. I'd join him on the sofa, wordlessly enjoying the music and soaring voices.

We were one of the lucky ones to have a piano and occasionally he would play a piece from Giuseppe Verdi's popular "Il Trovatore," with its plot full of kidnapping, beheading, burning babies, and bloody revenge. Perhaps it was his way of crying out, like the last line of the opera, "I am still alive!"

Listening to him play and watching him lose himself in the music left a powerful impression on me. From those moments, music became an essential presence in my life, as basic as air and water. Church, with its hymns in Latin and English, was a great pleasure.

We had an old windup Victrola and a small collection of recordings. By the time I became a teenager in the 1940s, the raw materials to make records were being diverted to wartime uses, so they were scarce. When I read in the newspaper one day that a large department store in Toronto had just received a big shipment, I was determined to have one and hitchhiked to Toronto, sixty miles away, to buy my first album, a copy of the Nutcracker Suite.

I played the Nutcracker over and over, driving everyone else in the house batty. My mother reached her limit with my next purchase – Ravel's Bolero, with its relentless military drumbeat. She'd come into the living room wringing her hands in exaggerated despair. "Ma, non spici mai?!" "Will it never end?!"

ooooo

As Dominic took charge of the family business, my mother took over my father's role as head of the house. When I was old enough to understand what she'd lived through, I began to see her as a remarkable person. By the time I went to medical school, I realized how amazing her life had been.

She'd given birth to sixteen children, and watched six of them die before the age of six. Most were taken by whatever disease was sweeping through the town in that pre-antibiotic era, but one of the tragedies was a result of a dreadful mishap. A nurse had placed a hot water bottle wrapped in a towel in the crib with my mother's latest newborn. The towel slipped off and the rubber bottle burned the child so badly that she died a few days later.

My mother told me this story later, recalling that the poor nurse was more distraught than she, who had by then become familiar with the fragility of life. She said she comforted the nurse, assuring her that the accident had been "Dio lo vuole" – God's will.

My mother believed just about everything was "God's will." "Dio lo vuole" slipped off her tongue frequently, no matter how terrible or trivial life's twists and turns. If someone died, it was God's will. If there was an earthquake, tsunami, conflagration, tornado, flood, deluge, or drought, my mother declared it God's will. If thousands of people died in a famine because they failed to prepare, God's hand was at work.

She also believed fervently in the power of prayer to shape God's will. During a family trip to Italy before I was born, my year-old brother Pacifico came down with a high fever. The Italian doctor who examined him warned my parents that the child was likely to die before they could get back to America.

My mother prayed to St Anthony, regarded by many Italians as the saint of miracles, all the way across the Mediterranean Sea and the Atlantic Ocean. She struck a bargain with St Anthony – if Pacifico survived, she would sew up a little Franciscan robe outfit, like the one St Anthony is usually depicted wearing, and make the boy wear it for two years.

My brother survived and my mother kept her end of the bargain – the brown robe was all he wore until he was three. I heard this story when I ran across old pictures of him dressed up like a tiny monk.

The phrase, "Dio lo vuole," found its way into my vocabulary as well, like a melody you can't get out of your head. But I reserved it for the most significant occasions. When I began to study the science of the human body, I realized that my mother was on to something.

The act of murder, for example, is the result of a chain of interactions in the brain. They may arise from real or imagined slights that, in a moment of madness or anger or confusion – temporary insanity – cause a breakdown in God's temple: the human mind. If we are created by God, as I believe, then God has introduced a potential chemical, neurological, or other defect and the resulting tragedy can be said to be His will. In becoming a doctor, I embraced the idea that the laws of physics and chemistry were put in effect by a creator, whether by fiat or evolution.

My mother's deep faith and observance saved her from succumbing to her sorrows. She devoted her spare time to charity, helping the needy, sick, and poor and she prayed at the drop of a hat. Tragic news, whether delivered by a neighbor or broadcast over the radio, would immediately elicit a prayer for the alternating assistance of God, Jesus, Mary, Joseph, or combinations thereof, depending on the enormity of the misfortune.

She kept her prayer book and rosary beads with her at all times. Whenever she took a moment to rest from making soup, cleaning, doing the wash, and her other household chores, she'd pick up her prayer book or finger her beads and say a few prayers. Every wall and flat surface sported pictures, carvings, or statues of Jesus, Mary, Joseph, and assorted saints. My parents' bedroom was shrine-like with fresh flowers and flickering lights from small glass oil lamps that gave off a slight odor of incense. She kept a large jar of spare oil to keep the lamps full and the wicks burning twenty-four hours a day.

The most striking picture in their bedroom was a life-sized painting of St George slaying the dragon. The creature had a long sinuous tail with a spiked tip and a terrifying man-like head with horns and fierce beady eyes. Hovering above the beast was St George, mounted on his horse, his lance raised as he prepared to administer the *coup de grace*. The devil's arms were raised in a desperate gesture to ward off the inevitable blow. To my childish eyes it was a truly terrifying depiction of good versus evil.

I had many hours to contemplate it when I was eight and came down with scarlet fever. My parents' room became the quarantine ward and I was confined to their bed. The customary treatment at the time called for letting the fever run its course. I spent agonizing days deathly ill with fever, sore throat, and rash, followed by the nasty spectacle of my skin coming off in shards.

For my convalescence, I became the centerpiece of my mother's cluttered shrine, the scent of burning oil in my nostrils, waking from awful, feverish dreams about the scary dragon-man. I rejoiced when the fever broke and I could escape.

CHAPTER TWO

JUSTICE AND INJUSTICE

The nuns at Sacred Heart Roman Catholic School in Guelph would all have ended up behind bars had they been judged by today's standards. In the 1940s, justice – and often injustice – was swift, cruel, and socially accepted, even for the youngest child. Many of us kids at Sacred Heart were first-generation Italian-Canadians who were painfully familiar with the whack of wooden spoons across the tops of our heads when we did something that displeased our harried mothers.

My first encounter with parochial discipline came like a thunderclap. I was an athletically precocious six-year-old who had discovered the thrill of banister sliding and stair leaping. A long staircase connected the first and second floors, interrupted by a landing. Like a young foal kicking up its heels, I found I could fly down the stairs by leaping three steps at a time. This required good foot-eye coordination in order to land precisely on the target step and be able to push off for another leap by holding on to the rail with my left hand.

I was sailing right along, intent on hitting my marks, got through the landing, and prepared for the last leap to the first floor. I had just launched myself from the banister when I sensed a dark presence in my periphery. For a split-of-a-split second, I saw a hand, palm facing me, sweeping with alarming speed toward my head. SMACK! The blow sent me sprawling across the hallway floor, through an open classroom door.

My head spun and my left ear roared. My focus slowly returned and I looked up into the grim scowl and bared teeth of Sister Monica. "RICHARD! You're to walk in the hallways, never run. Let this be a lesson to you."

"Yes, Sister," I muttered. My face blazed from the impact, and the shame.

Sacred Heart was just a half-block or so down Alice Street from our house. The strict discipline was part of the culture that made the school a beacon of faith for our struggling, aspirational community. I hoped my pious mother wouldn't find out what I'd done. Misbehaving at school reflected on the whole family. Whenever she found out we kids had been punished at school, we got a second dose at home, guilty or not.

The nuns who taught us always wore their black and white habits with starched white fronts and floor-length black gowns. From their corded belts hung a menacing leather strap they used to run a tight ship. We kids learned from day one that to keep the leather straps attached to their belts we would have to play by the rules. There would be no exceptions.

Justice – arrest, trial, conviction, sentencing, and punishment – was doled out on the spot for transgressions such as talking when you should have been silent, being silent when you'd been told to speak, running when you should have been walking, shoving in line, and so on. The strap was applied to the small, outstretched hands of errant children.

Girls, less rambunctious and considered more fragile, were seldom strapped. I found my chances to test the rules and experienced the searing burn and throb of bruised palms. The tougher boys did their best to deny the nuns any satisfaction or sense of victory by smiling throughout their strappings. On more than one occasion, the nun gave up.

On the other hand, I had a cousin who broke down and wailed before the nun had even taken her strap in hand, falling to his knees to beg for forgiveness and commutation of his sentence, refusing to produce his palms. This groveling infuriated the teacher, who proceeded to flog the child about the shoulders and arms, which made him howl even louder. Sensing she had gone too far, the sister stopped and returned to her desk, leaving my sobbing cousin on the floor to contemplate his humiliation.

This Dickensian episode would provoke official and parental outrage today, but in the 1930s and 1940s we kept our complaints to ourselves lest we risk a second thrashing at home. The idea of second-guessing a priest and or a nun was ludicrous. They were infallible and if one of the sisters thought you merited punishment, that was good enough for our parents.

One of the other episodes that stands out involved the punishment of a slightly older boy who'd been held back in our grade several years in a row for poor marks. He'd been caught playing hooky and – sin of sins – smoking cigarettes. A truant officer apprehended him and took him home. His exasperated mother dragged him off to school, knowing he'd face a much more terrifying fate than anything she might dish out.

I was sitting in class when this older boy's deep-throated screams filled the hallways, followed by the thumping of his heels striking the risers as he was dragged backwards up the stairs. Then we could hear him being hustled, still protesting, into the long, narrow cloakroom behind the classroom, followed by the violent smacking sound of the strap, and more howling. Some of the girls began to whimper.

Our teacher told us kids to bow our heads and pray to God to help Steve see the error of his ways. It was a brutal moment that stayed with me the rest of my life, in part because a few years later this young man committed suicide.

ooooo

Sacred Heart Church was the focal point of Alice Street, where parishioners came for healing of all sorts of problems, from financial distress, a drunken husband, and often physical disabilities. Sundays the church was packed, standing room only. The crippled and the sickly would find their way into the church pews or sat in their wheelchairs in the back. I often raised my head during prayers to sneak a look at the faces of the congregants and drink in the energy and intensity of their fervent pleas for deliverance from whatever misfortune had befallen them.

Tommy Balconi was a local bootlegger who'd been a large, overweight man until he came down with cancer and showed up at church emaciated. He shuffled down the aisle on his knees, in abject supplication. I prayed for him but soon after read his obituary in the paper.

Mrs Anna half sat, half kneeled in her pew, fingering her rosary beads, all the while quaking from a form of Parkinsonism. I prayed for her, too – that her suffering on earth would be short.

Even my father sometimes prayed aloud in audible fervor, though I could never understand his rapid-fire Italian. I wondered if all those prayers were ever answered. Although I could sense the fury and suffering in those lives, at that young age I was oblivious to real misery. My time would come but, mercifully, we are unable to foresee the future.

ooooo

My mother did all the cooking for the family, except on Sunday when my father prepared spaghetti and meatballs, the Sunday dinner staple and the main dish at Christmas, Easter, and Thanksgiving. We never saw a ham or a turkey when I was growing up.

While I did my homework, father would take over the kitchen. Still in his black tie, white shirt, and vest, he assembled spices, meats, fresh herbs, sauce, and pasta, preparing the meal with the finesse of a scientist conducting a chemistry experiment. He endlessly tested, tasted, and stirred with all the care and diligence of a master chef. It was hard to concentrate on my assignments on an empty stomach with bursts of heavenly aromas – garlic, carmelizing onions, and browning meat – filling the house. I eagerly awaited the magic moment when my father would extract a single strand of pasta from the steaming pot, nibble it, and call out "Al dente!"

CHAPTER THREE

THE FORTUNATE DISASTER

Most of the houses on Alice Street had porches or verandas and these were almost always occupied in warm weather by neighbors who were characters in the play called Alice Street.

Mr Ferraro was an old, heavyset man who spoke in a booming voice and sat on his porch fingering his rosary beads, his lips moving in silent prayer. I would wave to him and he always waved back.

Mrs Ferraro was short and could barely see over the porch railing. Whenever someone passed, she'd lift herself up on the arms of her chair and crane to see who it was, then sit down again.

Mrs Dupuis seldom smiled as she sat on her porch waving her ever-present fan. I imagined that her dourness reflected some painful secret.

Mr Skoronski liked to sit out in the direct sun, even on hot days. He was always neatly dressed and always wore a fedora.

A lone railroad spur in the neighborhood led to the place where the engineer drove the roundhouse locomotive each night, opened a hatch in the belly, and emptied the firebox onto the ground. It left behind a pile of glowing embers and spent clinkers. As soon as the engine left, people from the neighborhood would show up with their coal scuttles and tongs to pluck any usable lumps of coal. There was often a pile of fresh coal on top of the embers, which was like finding money laying on the ground. I would later learn that the engineer, who was known in the neighborhood as a friendly and compassionate man, had probably shoveled fresh coal into the firebox just before dumping the ashes. Everyone knew someone who needed a helping hand.

As poor as some of our neighbors were, tidiness was an obsession, especially among the local businessmen. For them, sweeping was more than the application of a broom to a surface. It seemed to be an art form and each had his own technique.

As an adult I became convinced that for these men sweeping was a symbolic cleansing of the psychological debris in their lives. Their castles might be modest, but they were still kings and still had the power to impose order.

My Uncle Joe was a professional sweeper at the Gilson factory, which manufactured its own brand of stoves and washing machines. Uncle Joe's job at Gilson was to keep the floor clear of metal debris. On the home front, he'd nurse a pipe between his teeth and sweep his steps with slow, deliberate strokes, cleaning the area with calculated precision. When he was finished he'd lean on his broom, pull deeply on his pipe, and expel a big cloud of blue smoke, surveying his workmanship with satisfaction.

Mike Sorbara, who lived across the street from us, swept as though driven by some invisible force. Every day he started at one end of his veranda, worked his way toward the top step, then down the steps to the walkway parallel to the lawn, and then the sidewalk. Finally, with one measured stroke, he would sweep the dirt, which was little more than a puff of dust since he did it every day, into the gutter.

My Uncle Vincent, the Alice Street cobbler, lived next door to us, so I often observed him as he swept with silent fury, as if scrubbing evil from the ground. Sweat would drip from his brow onto his cobbler's apron.

It was with Uncle Vincent that I had my first close encounter with the fragility of life. I was sitting outside one day when

Yvette Piquette, a young woman who lived across the street with her family, came flying out of her house, leaving the door wide open. She ran across the street into Uncle Vincent's shop. My uncle was hammering a nail into a sole when Yvette burst in screaming, waving and pointing across the street at the Piquette family house.

Uncle Vincent ran out of his shop still wearing his apron, gripping the bulges of nails in the pockets to keep the contents from flying out. Curious, I followed them into the Piquette home where I found my uncle kneeling on the floor over Mrs Piquette's lifeless body.

He gently moved her arms to see if she was conscious, but no response. He tried a crude version of resuscitation, pausing now and then to cross himself. Yvette was on the telephone, hysterical, calling for an ambulance in a mix of Canadian French and broken English. It arrived in short order and Uncle Vincent and Yvette moved out of the way while the medics tried to resuscitate Mrs Piquette.

"Coronary, I'll bet," one of the men said.

With the medical emergency out of his hands, Uncle Vincent's attention was drawn to a high pitched din that was growing louder. It was coming from his shop.

"Oh, my God!" he cried. "The motor."

He'd run out of the shop forgetting that he'd left on the motor that drove a series of belts that powered all his equipment for polishing and cutting leather. He ran back to his shop, from one crisis to another, holding up his apron like a lady gathers a long dress to keep from tripping.

The motor needed an operator to control the speed. Without anyone on the brake, the system accelerated until the long leather belts flew off their pulleys, which reduced the resistance even more. The motor was screaming and the floor was shaking so much the large glass window in the front was vibrating and seemed in imminent danger of shattering. Uncle Vincent managed to pull the shut-off switch just in time.

The medics stopped by Uncle Vincent's shop with a sobbing Yvette to report what we suspected: Mrs Piquette had passed away. Uncle Vincent, who often sang hymns while he worked, immediately genuflected and mouthed a silent prayer.

A hearse came and carried Mrs Piquette away, accompanied by Yvette. Uncle Vincent was subdued as he rethreaded all the belts back onto the pulleys. Then he closed shop and I went with him to his house next door. He sat down at the kitchen table, poured himself a glass of wine, and mumbled a few prayers. My aunt sat quietly in the chair beside him. None of us spoke.

My mother was waiting for me on the front porch when I got home. She had seen the hearse come and go. I told her the sad story. She listened, stroking the curls on my head. Then she sighed. "Dio lo vuole."

ooooo

I was an eager worker as a child, always willing to do chores at home or at the store. Inspired by my observations of everyone else's sweeping techniques, I enjoyed experimenting with ways to do my chores better. My sister-in-law Lola, Dominic's wife, once asked me to rake up the cut grass from the yard behind the store. I was seven years old. I went right to work and in no time had a nice tidy pile of dry grass cuttings. But it was a windy day and the grass was starting to blow around, messing up my hard work.

Behind the store next to the yard was a garage that housed a Model "T" Ford. I decided to scoop up the grass pile and carry it into the garage to get it out of the wind. I was proud of my ingenuity. The pile sat there undisturbed while the wind whipped beyond the corner of the garage.

The next challenge was to get rid of the grass. Everyone burned their leaves in the fall so that seemed like the grownup thing to do. I got some kitchen matches, ran back to the garage, and set the grass on fire.

A few wisps of smoke curled up at first and everything seemed to going just fine until the smoldering suddenly burst into a pillar of flames. The gravity of the situation sank in slowly until the tarpaper nailed to the bare-wood walls ignited. The flames raced up the wall and licked at the rafters.

I panicked. My sole thought was to run home, down the street from the store. I barreled through our front door just as the first sirens sounded. I bounded up the stairs to the third-floor attic where I scrambled over to the attic window in time to see a couple of fire trucks roaring down the street.

It was wash day and my aunt sometimes dried the clothes on lines in the attic. She had heard the racket and came up to investigate.

"Richie, what in God's name is all this stomping around. Where have you been?" Another fire truck wailed past on the street below. She walked over to the window and bent over to peer out. "What's happening with all this commotion? What's going on around here?"

"Nothing. I wasn't doing anything." My face and neck burned. She flashed me a frown, then went back downstairs.

I sat in the attic, hugging my knees, my stomach churning. I was in the biggest trouble of my life. I was the condemned man waiting for the clang of the prison door that signaled the guards had come to drag me off to the guillotine.

It took about a half hour, and the clang took the form of the deep, commanding voice of my brother Silvio, the doctor, resonating through the floorboards.

"WHERE IS RICHIE?!"

I descended the stairs with shoulders slumped and wobbly knees to find with Silvio with a man in a bulky fireman's jacket and a stony look in his eyes.

"Richie, what the dickens did you do at the store? The neighbors saw you raking grass and the next thing the garage burns down."

I confessed through tears of shame and humiliation. The fireman took notes on his pad. As I told the story, the look on his face softened. I must have cut quite a pathetic figure, hiccup-crying as I tried to explain how I just wanted to be helpful.

Silvio shook his head, but I could see a flicker of gentleness in his eyes.

"You know you're not to play with matches. Now you go back there and you'll see why."

No sentence was imposed. Not even a smack on the head. But I didn't need it. I was doing a good job of punishing myself.

The destruction stunned me. The garage and car had been reduced to a pile of charred debris. Borghesi's barn next door, which housed two cows and several months' worth of hay stored for the winter months, had burned to the ground. All that remained was smoking embers. The back of the store and the back of Borghesi's house bore scorch marks. I worried that there was an axe awaiting me, but none ever fell. I received my fire-safety lecture, but beyond that it seemed I had been found innocent of malice, and guilty only of good-intentioned, childish bumbling.

The incident was never spoken of again and it would be forty years before I learned why, serendipitously. On a visit home, I ran into a cousin who was an insurance agent in town. We chatted and he happened to bring up the garage fire, lowering his voice in a conspiratorial tone. Even after all those years, my shame was so close to the surface that I braced myself for a reprimand.

"Richie, you have no idea what a wonderful thing you did for your family, burning down those garages."

"Huh?"

"Everybody knew it was just a dumb little kid accident. But nobody made a fuss about it so the insurance would pay off. It was the middle of the Depression, remember?

"Your little fire paid for both garages, the car, and the damage to the back of the store and house. Those settlement checks came just at the right time. You never knew it, but you did a wonderful thing for both families!"

CHAPTER FOUR

MY **SECOND ENCOUNTER** WITH **DEATH**

Victoria Day, 24 May 1939, a holiday celebrating the birth of Queen Victoria 120 year earlier, fell on a Wednesday, which meant we kids had the day off from school. But we had to go to a special morning mass – I particularly had to be there because I was an altar boy. Some of my friends were altar boys as well, and that day I shared my duties with three of them: Massimo, Duke, and Duke's older brother Manny.

It was a warm spring day and we were fidgety to get out into it as Father O'Brien emerged from the sanctuary and began the service: "I will go before the altar of God," to which we replied, "To God who giveth joy to my youth."

When it was finally over, we peeled off our surplice and soutane, hung them neatly, and headed up to the dam on the Speed River where there was a park and a lake. A deep race ran beside the dam and was opened to keep the river from flooding during the spring melt. In summer, the race still had enough water in it to make it a popular diving spot and swimming hole.

We sat on the grass on a promontory that separated the dam from the race and watched the older kids dive from the bridge. We spent most of the day there, hanging out, talking to the other kids, and enjoying the warm sun.

When we decided to go home, Manny in his bright yellow shirt was nowhere to be found. We searched all the usual places, then extended our hunt across the bridge to the other side of the dam.

From the bridge we had a clear view of the water below the dam. Duke noticed first, pointing and crying out, "What's that?" There, in the shallow depths of a large pool of water, there appeared to be the outline of a figure, sprawled in the water, wearing a bright yellow shirt.

We raced to the end of the dam and scrambled down to the river's edge, but we couldn't reach Manny and the water was too deep for us kids. Duke dashed off toward home crying and screaming for his father. Massimo and I sprinted into a nearby building and blurted to the first adult we saw, an old man, "Our friend is under the water! Hurry!"

The man followed us outside. He tore off his suit jacket and vest and waded out into the river, stretching to grab hold of Manny, who was floating face down in the deepest part. He turned him over and towed him back, labouring against the deep water. At the water's edge we helped pull Manny's limp body out onto a ledge. The man began artificial respiration. Massimo and I watched, stupefied by the horror, trembling with fear. Manny couldn't be dead, could he?

A fire rescue truck came wailing up to the edge of the dam, and the crew scuttled with their equipment down to the waterfront to take over. Duke returned with his frantic father who, upon seeing his boy's body sprawled out on the concrete, burst into uncontrollable sobs. A hard lump formed in my throat.

A growing crowd stood around in sober silence as the firemen worked on Manny. After ten minutes they stopped, bowed their heads for a moment, and radioed for the coroner. Manny's father collapsed. Massimo and I were ordered to our homes, where our frantic parents had already heard the awful news. My mother wanted to know how such a thing could have happened with so many people around.

The next day our teachers were somber. Some were red-eyed and dabbed at their cheeks with their handkerchiefs. Manny had been well-liked, always courteous and soft-spoken. His death was felt deeply by all, each in his or her own way.

I was deeply depressed for a week, even though I had gazed upon more than my share of bodies lying in caskets. As an altar boy I was often called on to sing the traditional funeral hymn, the "Dies Irae" (Day of Wrath), at requiem masses. The first verse was,

Dies irae! dies illa
Solvet saeclum in favilla
Teste David cum Sibylla!

which translates roughly as:

Day of wrath! O day of mourning!
See fulfilled the prophets' warning,
Heaven and earth in ashes burning!

We altar boys sang in the choir at Manny's funeral at Sacred Heart before an overflow crowd. His death evoked the sympathy of many mothers and fathers who harbored unspoken terrors of finding themselves in the same situation as Manny's parents. I'm sure every one thought, There but for the grace of God ...

The coffin was smothered in flowers whose perfume mingled with the candle smoke and permeated the church. Sitting there quietly waiting for the service to begin, I watched large waxen tears slide slowly down the candle into the receptacle below. The only sound were stifled sobs in the pews.

Suddenly the organ broke into a hymn and Father O'Brien, with his retinue, came out into the sanctuary to begin the funeral mass. He faced the altar, raised his arms to Heaven, and intoned in a deep sonorous voice, "I will go unto the altar of God," and once more – but without Manny's voice – we replied in an almost incomprehensible whisper, "To God who giveth joy to my youth."

ooooo

The following summer I got a surprise invitation from Father O'Brien to attend Camp Brebeuf, a new Catholic summer camp for boys in the woods near Rockwood, a small town about seven miles from Guelph. It was named forSaint Jean de Brebeuf the Jesuit missionary who was tortured to death by the Iroquois Indians in 1649.

The surprise was that I could go for free, which was the only thing that made it possible. My mother gave me permission and I excitedly drove to camp with Father O'Brien, taking a basic kit of toothbrush, towel, and change of clothing. We arrived in the dark and after I had been assigned to my bunk, I said my prayers and added thanks to God for letting me go to camp.

The next morning after breakfast, while all the other kids were getting organized for volleyball, basketball, and soccer, I was pulled aside with a handful of the other boys. "This morning," the counselor said, "we're going to clean the Bishop's cabin that he uses each weekend." It suddenly dawned on me how I was able to go to camp: I was paying my way with labour. No one ever came out and said it, but the quid pro quo was clear. I was given a broom and vacuum cleaner and put to work. The other boys cleaned the kitchen, some dusted, some collected and took out garbage.

After lunch, we charity cases got to participate in sports with the paying clientele and then back to dinner and bed. I was happily exhausted that night.

The next day was a repeat, except the job that morning was to empty the "honey buckets" – the latrine pails. The latrine was built on a hillside, and you entered on the uphill side. Inside was a long bench with a series of holes where you sat to do your business, into those pails. On the downhill side were compartments with doors that we were to open and remove the pails.

The other boys and I who'd been assigned this detail had to carry those buckets – some retching from the smell and all trying to avoid splashing ourselves – down to a deep trench carved by a tractor. Once the buckets had been emptied into the trench, the mess was covered with a layer of earth.

After breakfast the next day, our counselor told us, "Today we're going to the stream that runs through camp." My heart leaped for joy. I would get a chance to go swimming! Then he added, "We're going to be building a swimming hole."

This proved to be hard labor. The riverbed was shale, which we had to break with a crowbar. When then dislodged the pieces, which were large and heavy, and carried them to the riverbank, where the counselor, who did no work, gave us an encouraging word, commenting from time to time how the riverbed was getting deeper and soon it would be deep enough to swim. I felt like an Egyptian slave boy hauling stones for the Pharaoh's pyramid, or a prisoner on a chain gang.

After dinner that night I found a telephone, called my parents, and asked them to come get me.

"What's wrong, Richie?" Mother asked. "Don't you like the other boys?"

I didn't tell her I had been Shanghaied. I just told her I was homesick and unhappy. My aunt picked me up the next morning and I breathed a sigh of relief as the car rolled down the dusty lane. I had escaped.

My working life, however, was just beginning.

One of my early chores in the family store was to help the woman who came to scrub the floors on Sundays, when it was closed. The Ontario climate being snowy so much of the year, the floor planks quickly became black with cinders and soot from the streets and sidewalks. Beck, as she called herself, was an elderly, black woman who wore long, heavy dresses and a scarf. She rested her knees on a jute sack and wore thick, black, rubber gloves to protect her hands from the lye soap flakes she'd scatter before she began to scour with a large bristle brush.

When the pail of water got dirty, she'd send me outside to pour it out, rinse the pail, and refill it with fresh water. While I did this, she rested, lighting up a corn cob pipe and taking a few puffs.

When she had worked her way from one end of the store to the other, the wooden floor had been restored to its pristine condition. Beck would put her hands on her hips and declare, "It's as black as Toby's rear-end." I never learned who Toby was.

In August 1939, after my tenth birthday, my big brother Dominic, who ran the grocery store, sat me down, looked me in the eye, and announced, "I am going to get you a bicycle."

My first bike! I had a few seconds of unadulterated joy. Then he said, "This is going to be a special bicycle, custom made. It will have a sturdy kickstand to hold it up when it's parked, a specially built carrier to deliver groceries, and an electric generator for the tail light, so you can deliver groceries at night.

"Now the bike costs $42." That was a staggering amount of money. "You'll start working in the store after school and on weekends, to help support the family. I'll pay you $1.10 every Saturday morning. Out of that $1.10 you're going to take a dollar each week to Mr Chapman at the bike shop for forty-two weeks until the bicycle is paid off. You can keep the ten cents for yourself."

When I told my mother, I discovered she'd been in on it all along.

"Now that you're making money," she said, "it's time you start tithing. You save a nickel every week for the church poorbox. The nickel left over you can keep to do with as you please."

Thus, at the age of ten I had officially become an indentured servant, $42 in debt. But I soon grew accustomed to working in the family business. The presumption that youngsters should contribute to the family's welfare was immigrant thinking and this sort of arrangement has fallen out of fashion. But it did teach me business skills at an early age.

One of my chores was restocking the potato display in the middle of the store, which required lugging heavy sacks of spuds. By the end of each week, I had acquired a pile of empty potato sacks, along with many bushel baskets that had held vegetables and fruits on display in the front of the store. There were also left-over baskets in which meat had been delivered.

I quickly discovered that the empty sacks could be sold for three cents each at the Guelph Farmer's Market downtown, and that the baskets would fetch a nickel. So every Saturday morning, before work, I would lash the sacks and baskets to my wagon and, holding the cargo with one hand to keep it from toppling over, I'd trudge the two miles up the hill to the center of town.

My best customer was an elderly lady in a neck-to-ankles leather apron who sold meat and vegetables from her farm. She always examined the sacks or jute bags for holes. When she found one, she'd say, "Oh my! This one has a hole. I'll have to repair it so it's only worth 2 cents."

There were about a dozen sacks in the pile each week, and I noticed that she only looked at the ones on the top and then flipped the pile to look at one or two on the bottom. After that I hid the sacks with holes in the middle of the pile.

My revenue from this weekly trip averaged about a dollar, which I turned over to my mother for safekeeping. Occasionally I would use the money to buy a live Plymouth Rock hen from one of the farmers to take home. My mother would ooh and aah and praise me for choosing such a nice fat hen.

My mother kept pinned to the inside of her dress the key to the locked drawer in the buffet in the dining room where she kept important papers and an envelope with my name on it and my sack and basket money inside. From time to time she'd sit me down at the dining room table and explain – in a hushed tone reserved for grave, grownup matters – that there had been a crisis that required dipping into my earnings and swallowed up months worth of work dragging that wagon four miles every Saturday morning.

Being the dutiful son, I was always glad to help out. When Pacifico returned from Europe after serving in the army during the Second World War, he went to school in London, Ontario, to study electronics. He had a government subsidy under the Veteran's Education Bill, but my mother told me that sometimes he didn't have enough money for food. This upset me and she said, "You know, you have twenty dollars saved in the drawer. Could we send this to Pacifico?" With enthusiasm and pride, I blurted, "Yes! Send it right away."

It would be sixty years before I learned from Pacifico that he never received the money. He assured me that he had been well taken care of by the Veteran's Education Bill.

Where the money went I can only speculate. Donating to light candles at church was one of my mother's favorite pastimes, along with money to baptize pagan babies in far off lands. And when any of my many siblings came to visit, she'd always send them home with a little money she'd surreptitiously tucked into their palms.

Whenever I used my money to buy something special, like the chicken, my mother made sure I got the first serving. When I showed up one Saturday up with a chocolate rabbit, she gave me the usual praise, and added a big hug and a kiss. Then she told me that my ninety-nine-year-old grandfather in Italy loved chocolate. "He would love to have this rabbit, don't you think?"

I was dumbstruck. I'd never met any of my grandparents, and I felt no obligation to give up that chocolate rabbit. But I kept my selfish thoughts to myself and watched in wistful silence as she put it in a empty cloth sugar bag, sewed it shut, and packed it in a box with paper to keep it from being broken. The parcel was then mailed to Italy.

I consoled myself that it was God's will that I should never enjoy so much as a nibble of that rabbit. But in a twist of fate, it was apparently also God's will that my ninety-nine-year-old grandfather would eat too much of the chocolate, suffer an adverse reaction, and die shortly thereafter.

ooooo

School was where I was happiest and in fifth grade I had a lay teacher, Miss Phelan, who noticed my enthusiasm for answering every question and my interest in animals. She moved my seat next to a bookshelf that served as the classroom library.

She, like myself, loved the natural world. She lived on a farm on the outskirts of Guelph and one autumn day took the entire class to a local forest area for a nature lesson. The leaves had turned and the trees were busy with squirrels gathering nuts. I was in Heaven. Miss Phelan must have noticed because when we got back to school, she took the time to show me "Bedtime Stories" by Thornton Burgess, a conservationist from Cape Cod who wrote thousands of stories and 170 books for children about the beauty of nature.

I dove in and became transfixed, ignoring the recess bell to stay in the classroom so I could continue to read. Miss Phelan insisted I go outside and get some exercise. "But if you want, you can take the books home and read them at night."

I made short work of the series, polishing off one a night. When I got to the last one, I asked her if she had any more. She told me I would find many more at the Guelph Public Library, including Burgess' more advanced books like "Old Mother West Wind." Each volume explained an aspect of nature and its creatures: "Why Grandfather Frog Has No Tail," and "Birds You Should Know."

I was anxious to read through this new set of books and after class ran to the library to get my card. When the librarian noticed my home address – 51 Alice Street – she frowned.

"Do you have a brother named Mike?"

I did, I said.

"Well, he borrowed a book a few years ago and never returned it. He owes the library a dollar and I can't let you take out any books until that's paid.

I turned to my mother, but she sent me on to Dominic who, having dealt with Mike's forgetfulness before, threw up his hands and cried out, "When will it end?"

But he gave me the dollar, and I returned home that day with my first *Mother West Wind* book. My education in anatomy and the nature of life had begun in earnest.

CHAPTER FIVE

LESSONS ABOUT MONEY

My eighth grade teacher was Sister Monica, the same nun who'd sent me sprawling when I was leaping down the stairs in first grade. I tread cautiously that year, applied myself, and ended the year with the highest grade point average among the boys. This won me an award from the Parish Ladies Auxiliary, given at a school ceremony.

The president of the auxiliary said a few words and handed me a check while the audience applauded. I thanked everyone and walked tall all the way back to the store, where I proudly showed Dominic the check. It was for $25! That was equal to a hundred miles of trudging back and forth with my potato sacks and baskets.

Dominic's brows arched as he eyed the check. Then he said in a solemn tone, as both he and my mother often did when discussing my money, "You realize that next year you are going to need money for books when you go to high school. So why don't you give me the check, and I will hold the money for you until you start high school in September." It seemed logical so I gave him the check, having had it in my possession for all of thirty minutes.

My mother agreed with Dominic and I took it on faith that the two of them were working as a team to see that I learned the rudiments of economics early in life. The lesson, however, would not become clear until I was older.

My friends and I spent the summer discussing and debating the big choice we would have to make in September: whether to take the industrial or the academic program. I sought Dominic's counsel and he recommended that I learn a trade. With my good grades, the academic route would inevitably lead to the opportunity to attend university and that was expensive, he said. As an electrician, I could begin earning a good living after just three years of study.

So I dutifully enrolled in the industrial program. I disassembled a car engine, worked on a lathe, built wooden furniture, and wired a miniature house. Toward the end of the first year, my brother, Mike, who had earned a teaching degree in college and played professional football, came home for a visit. When he found out I had enrolled in the industrial program, he scowled.

"Whatever possessed you to do that?" he asked.

His apparent disapproval caught me off guard.

"Dominic said I should, because then I wouldn't have to worry about having enough money to go to university."

Mike flew out of the chair and stormed out of the house, headed for the store. I tagged along at some distance and hung back as Mike chastised Dominic for steering me away from the college prep program.

Dominic was equally vociferous. "Who's going to pay for it? I've suffered enough in this store, having to earn the money for you and Silvio to go to Western. I've done my share."

Mike prevailed by pointing out that, since I would have to start high school over again, this meant the first tuition payment was five years away – the usual four years of high school plus the customary college prep year of our British-influenced school system.

That fall I started high school all over again, in the academic program. I knew no one in my class but I rather liked the change. I loved the classes, excited to begin learning French, studying advanced math, reading Shakespeare, and all the rest. Mike's visit and advocacy of my behalf changed the course of my life in the most wonderful and profound way.

Silvio, who like Mike had been supported through college by my father and the store, also changed my life, but the circumstances were quite different. Silvio and Mike had been gifted athletes. Silvio had gone on to earn his medical degree from Western Ontario, and then opened his practice in Guelph. He had become a respected member of the community, the first non-anglo to be admitted to the Guelph Country Club. Everyone in town looked up to him. "See," as we in the family called him, was a stalwart presence in our lives, an authority figure whose deep, sonorous voice commanded attention and respect. He dropped by our house several times a week for lunch, always dressed in a crisply creased suit and a tie.

The invasion of Poland in September 1939, when I was ten years old, came just as Silvio was about to leave for Austria to do postdoctoral work in the latest surgical techniques. With that avenue closed to him, he returned to Guelph, disbanded his practice, and joined the Eastern Division of the Canadian Army Medical Corp. He spent most of his war service at the Canadian Forces Base in Valcartier, Quebec.

I rarely saw Silvio after he went into the army, and heard little about him until I was fourteen. One day in the spring of 1944, Dominic phoned our house and told me I was needed right away at the store. Silvio, he explained, was sick – so sick that my parents were leaving right away for London, Ontario, about seventy-five miles away, to be with him. In my parents' absence, I was to fill in at the store.

I hadn't heard anything about Silvio being ill, and the last time I'd seen him he appeared to be his usual hale and hearty self. The notion that he was gravely ill was hard to fathom. The Silvio I knew had, like my brother Mike, been a star football player in high school and in college. Both had made names for themselves, referred to in the local newspaper from time to time as the "Valeriote boys." There was nothing fragile about Silvio, so it was impossible to imagine him bed-ridden.

But, unknown to the family, he'd been diagnosed years earlier with Hodgkin's disease, a fatal form of lymphoma cancer. Only his wife, Velma, a nurse, and his two children knew about it. The disease had been in remission for nearly a decade. Now, suddenly, we learned not only that he had been sick but that he was on his death bed. Silvio's doctors had been treating him with chemotherapy and blood transfusions, but he had become so weak the treatments were abandoned and they were doing their best to keep him comfortable as he faded away.

While my parents were away tending to Silvio, I stayed out of school to help Dominic with the business. I assumed I would be back in school in a few days, but Silvio lingered for a month and my parents ended up staying in his house in London for the duration. I visited once or twice, but he was so sick we hardly talked beyond greetings and goodbyes. His skin had turned yellow and he was so emaciated my mother was able to pick him up. The change was shocking and heart-breaking.

Silvio was delivered from his suffering at the age of thirty-three on 2 May 1944. Most of Guelph turned out for the funeral, which included full military honors. In the days that followed, the radio in our home, which was such an important part of life during those war years, was silent. That year, for the first time, we had Christmas without a tree.

My mother again consoled herself that it had been God's will to take her seventh child. She accepted it with the same equanimity she had shown the nurse who scalded her baby years before. "God had a purpose for his early death," she told me.

"One day I will be reunited with him." From Silvio's death until her own many years later at age eighty-six, my mother wore only black.

Years later, in 1952, I learned fuller details of Silvio's medical history, purely by happenstance. I was married and earning my bachelor's degree at McGill University. A big snowstorm had fallen on the city and the buses weren't running and my wife, Polly, and I walked to school from our basement apartment in the Westmount neighborhood.

As we trudged through the drifts along Sherbrooke Street, both of us shivering from the cold, I decided to put out my thumb to see if some motorist would take pity on us. A car stopped, and we hopped in, introducing ourselves and explaining to the driver that I was finishing up my undergraduate studies and planned to go on to medical school.

The driver said he was going to McGill as well and introduced himself as Ray Lawson, a professor of surgery at McGill Medical School. Then he said, "Did you say Valeriote? That's an unusual name. I played football at Western with a guy named Valeriote."

"That was my brother!"

"For Heaven's sake. You're See's brother?!" I was stunned to hear a total stranger calling Silvio by his family nickname.

Dr Lawson said he had been the commander of See's army division when See signed up. Even the doctors had to go through an initial medical exam, so Lawson had known from the start about Silvio's diagnosis. That, he explained, was why he had assigned See to Valcartier instead of a more distant assignment.

CHAPTER SIX

MY ONE AND ONLY HUNTING LESSON

Between high school, homework, my duties at the store, and church, my time was fully booked. I wouldn't have dared complain, especially after my mother reassured me, "Some day you will go to college, and Dominic will pay for it just as the store paid for Silvio and Mike. Besides, you must do your share to help support the family." In fact I become indispensable, a jack of all trades.

One of my duties was to stop at several homes on the outskirts of Guelph on my drive home from high school to pick up grocery orders from families that were too poor to afford a car or a telephone. I sat on tattered davenports and at scarred kitchen tables, recording orders on scraps of paper that I turned over to Dominic for delivery the following day.

These were the homes of the working poor, and the experience of visiting them opened my eyes to a new world.

The father of one of these families worked at a local foundry and when I came to pick up the order, the bicycle he rode to and from the plant would be leaning on the railing of the front porch. He worked around blast furnaces and always returned home covered from head to toe with soot.

I would often find him sitting in the middle of the living room, neck-deep in a large wooden tub brimming with hot soapy water, his face black with soot except for clean rings around his eyes left by his goggles. As I sat taking down the list of groceries, his wife scrubbed her husband down and washed his hair.

Some of the items they ordered were the ingredients of "home brew," a beer made from hops, brown sugar, yeast, barley, and malt. While his wife scrubbed, he drank his after-work brew from a large bowl and then picked up a can of Daily Mail tobacco. With the expertise of a connoisseur, he rolled a cigarette, lit it, and exhaled a stream of smoke.

His daughter, in a crisp, clean pinafore, looked on with pride. As his wife worked, the rings around the man's eyes merged with his face, she combed his hair, and he sank to his neck in the warm water, his eyes closed in a look of pure serenity. Theirs was a hard life, but I was moved by the pride and love with which they lived it.

Back at the store I worked the counter, waiting on customers who were overwhelmingly immigrants from all over Europe. A Polish man came in every night at the same time to buy food for his supper. He was gregarious and taught me the Polish words for butter, cabbage, sausage, and tobacco and told me I was a "dobra chilawik" – a good boy.

He was so predictable you could set your clock by his visits. He came directly from the foundry, his clothes smelling of sweat and coal smoke. He spoke very few words of English, communicating in choppy, incomplete sentences and hand gestures. One evening after his shift, he didn't come. In a community store like ours, you noticed little things like that. I commented on it to Dominic.

He grabbed his coat off its hook and pulled it on. "He lives alone. I better look in on him." A short time later he returned with a long face and the news that he'd found the man sitting in an overstuffed chair, dead of an apparent heart attack.

This death struck me as especially sad. He had died alone at the end of a hard day's work, reminding me of Henry David

Thoreau's observation that, "The mass of humanity live out their lives in quiet desperation."

My father was living proof of this dismal outlook, and perhaps the contrast between his unhappy example and Silvio's indomitable spirit helped stoke my enthusiasm for life, learning, and healing. My father was often a ghostly presence in my life, but we had our moments.

I got my first hunting license the winter after I turned sixteen. There were no gun safety classes in those days so what I knew about firearms came from my father's single-shot, sixteen-gauge shotgun, a caliber somewhere between the weakest and the most powerful.

The day I came home with my license, I asked my father to take me hunting for rabbits. My father had been an avid hunter in his early life, but he was sixty-three by this time, retired and sedentary. It had been years since he'd gone hunting.

My mother overheard my request and, knowing my father would find any excuse to stay put and sulk rather than spend time tramping in the snow with me, jumped in immediately. She implored him, in Italian, to go out and spend some time with me. "You never do anything with Richie. Be a good father and take him hunting."

My father protested. He was tired. It was cold out. What was there to shoot in the middle of winter?

My mother persisted, periodically raising her hands in supplication, as if begging God to chime in on her side. To the uninitiated, they appeared to be bitter enemies going at it tooth and nail, with vigorous hand gestures and the harsh poetry of rapid-fire Italian.

But my mother was passionately laying out all the reasons why he should take me hunting and wearing my father out. Finally he threw up his hands in surrender and got dressed, pulling his overcoat on over his suit, white shirt, tie, and vest. He grumpily clapped his Fedora on his head, tromped upstairs, and came back down with the shotgun and a box of shells. He jerked his head toward the door and I followed him out of the house.

No one would have mistaken my father for a hunter, dressed the way he was. But I didn't care. I couldn't wait to bag my first game to bring home for my mother to cook.

The weather was bitter following a foot of fresh snow that had fallen during the night – terrible hunting conditions. But I was too wound up to notice. I had never held a shotgun before, and I was delighted when my father handed it to me, unloaded, to carry until we were out of town.

The city streets had been plowed but when we got to the outskirts we found the country roads were walled by six-foot drifts, making it impossible to strike out across a field looking for a rabbit or a pheasant. My father stopped and slid a shell into the barrel of the shotgun, snapped the barrel into position, and handed the weapon to me.

"Avanza," he muttered, gesturing for me to go ahead of him. "I follow. So you don't shoot me by mistake." That was the sum total of my hunting lesson. I stepped down the road and he trudged along, far behind. I held the gun the way I imagined I was supposed to, scanning the seamless white landscape for any sign of movement.

No creature stirred, not even a chickadee. No cars came driving by. The only sounds were the crunch of my shoes and the sighing of the wind in the pines alongside the road. It wasn't long before I heard my father grumbling and turned to see him throw up his hands. "Ma siamo pazzi!" he said. Crazy!

I walked back to him, handed over the gun, and he removed the shell. Then he handed the gun back, stuffed his hands in his pockets, and we walked home in silence, ice crystals forming on his mustache. He saved his complaints for my mother, who eagerly asked if we'd brought home the bacon, or rabbit. "Non vedemmo niente!" he said, shaking off his overcoat. "Nothing out there but two fools too stupid to stay home where it's nice and warm!"

It had been a rare, brief, laconic interaction, but over time it became a cherished memory.

Five years would pass before my father and I exchanged more than a few words. I was attending McGill University, studying textbook Italian, and decided one weekend to sit down and compose the first letter I ever wrote to my parents in their native language.

Within a week, I received a package containing razor blades, shaving lotion, and other toiletries, all of which I needed but were unaffordable. There were also some pepperonis, also a luxury, which tasted all the better for having come from my parents' store.

The biggest surprise in the package was a note from my then sixty-nine-year-old father, with the salutation, "Carissimo Figlio" – "Dearest Son." It was the first time in my life he had addressed me with such tenderness. In the next year, he wrote to me about a dozen times, always in response to my letters. His handwriting was elaborate, with flourishes that, since I had studied the language only in its published form, made the words difficult to decipher at times.

He and my mother always began by invoking God's name and asking His blessings on me, which was food for my spirit. Occasionally my father would slip in a dollar bill, a windfall to a starving student at a time when a dollar bought ten loaves of bread.

Pa's notes always ended with the admonition, "Mangiare, dormire, studiare, evitare gli eccessi." "Eat, sleep, study, avoid excess." The last was easy to obey. I had neither time nor money for anything resembling excess.

My brother Dominic – ever the hawk-eyed businessman and a penny-watching father with four children to feed – wrote to me during this period asking me to discourage Father from mailing me those care packages. "The postage costs 65 cents," he complained. "Pa should just send you the money, and you buy what you need in Montreal."

My father ignored Dominic and I never brought up the subject. I loved getting the packages, and it was clear Pa enjoyed preparing and sending them. Each letter he wrote was like unearthing buried treasure. They were short and contained no grand revelations, but they made me feel a direct connection with him that was tactile and new.

I would re-read them several times, studying the style of his script, comparing his Italian to the version I'd learned at McGill, trying to get to know him better. I kept them in a safe place with my other most-precious possessions.

Perhaps I had had a premonition. After a year of monthly letter-writing, he stopped responding. I missed the exchanges, but I knew my father well enough to guess that he'd slipped back into the low state that had haunted him for so many years.

CHAPTER SEVEN

MY MOTHER AND
MY FEET

My busy work life at the family store kept me occupied but never distracted me from earning consistently good marks. My height shot up to six feet and at 160 pounds I was lean, tall, and all the lifting at the store had made me strong. But I was still wet behind the ears about the ways of the real world.

One of the most jarring lessons came in eleventh grade, thanks to an elderly English teacher, Margaret MacFee. She was also my homeroom teacher and on the first day of school she announced, "I think that all the people in this classroom would like to know who their classmates are. Will all those who are not of English, Irish, or Scotch heritage please stand up."

Her request struck me as odd and intimidating. But I dutifully rose, along with a handful of other students who were Greek or Hungarian or who-knew-what. No sooner had she instructed us to sit back down when she asked those who were not Protestant to stand up. I rose along with a few other Catholics, a couple of Jewish kids, and one whose family was Greek Orthodox. A nervous titter ran through the room.

Nothing about this exercise felt good. Far from an acknowledgment of the wonderful diversity of our community, she seemed to be singling us non-anglos out for some sort of subversive humiliation. She never made the "English, Irish, or Scotch" kids stand up.

My distrust of Mrs MacFee faded as I got into the rhythm of the school year. I found all my classes easy and enjoyable. Everything seemed to be going along smoothly until one day in her English class, when she was handing out marked tests. She had handed out everyone else's and I was about to ask what happened to mine when she declared that she wanted to discuss a certain student's paper. It had to be mine. I gulped. "I want to discuss this paper since it was so unusual."

I had written a long dissertation on a poem, and I thought it was quite good and hoped she was going to commend me for my effort.

"This paper is one of the worst that I have ever seen," she began. My ears started to burn. She stood a few feet from my desk without looking at me, arms folded, the notorious test tucked in her fist.

"I had to give this student a failing grade. Now I certainly understand why he did so poorly. It was because of his ethnic background. He probably doesn't speak English at home and that's why he has trouble mastering the English language."

She stepped forward and thrust the creased paper at me with a grimace. My heart hammered against my ribs. A scarlet "38" was scrawled across the top of the first page. The paper seemed to be covered with red pencil stains.

A failing grade! I was horrified, mortified. It was the only failing grade I had ever received! My scalp crawled as a rush of adrenaline flooded my bloodstream. I stood to take the paper from her hand. She clucked, shook her head, and said archly to the room, "I'm sure that this young man probably does well in other subjects but finds English difficult."

I glared at her as a furnace of heat rose up my neck. For the first time, I saw in stark relief that Mrs MacFee was an old lady.

Her wrinkled, sagging skin had been slathered with a crust of cheap makeup. Her lips were covered with garish lipstick that looked like red grease, which had leached into the tiny wrinkles around her mouth like capillaries.

My ears roared. Her lips were moving but I couldn't make out a word. I had the strongest urge to strike out. Instead I stared down at the test paper in my hand, my breath coming in gulps.

The list of my answers to the test questions were all marked with red zeros. One question had been to define the word "hoar" as used in a line of a poem by Henry Wadsworth Longfellow. "The Warden of the Cinque Ports" had been written as a tribute to the Duke of Wellington when he died in 1852. The verse in question read:

He did not pause to parley or dissemble,
But smote the Warden hoar;
Ah! What a blow! That made all England tremble
And groan from shore to shore.

I had written "white haired, white bearded." A red "o" had been written over the answer. I knew I had the right answer and was going to protest, but first I stole a glance at the paper of the boy sitting next to me. His answer was the same as mine, but he had gotten a "2." The pattern appeared to repeat itself all the way down my paper.

Out of the fog of hurt and bewilderment, Mrs McAfee's voice floated back into focus. "... and I had to deduct fifteen marks just for punctuation. Dear, dear!"

I examined the test but could see no red marks for misspelling or incorrect punctuation. Then it seemed to hit her that I was on to her. She snatched the paper out of hands. "I'll review your test again to see if perhaps I might find some additional points."

I slumped into my seat, slack-jawed and trembling with frustration, rage, and humiliation. My classmates were trying their hardest to stare at me without looking. I stumbled out of class in a daze. None of it made any sense.

The incident had so disturbed others that by the end of classes it had become the scandal of the day. Tongues were wagging and even the teachers were casting sympathetic glances my way. Miss Garland, my French teacher, summoned me after class to advise me to request the paper back from Mrs MacFee the next day in class. "Then bring it to me and I'll have someone else read and re-grade it. I'm sure it's all a misunderstanding, Richard. Don't look so sad. Everything will be all right."

Bucked up by Miss Garland's kind words, the next day in English I presented myself to Mrs MacFee and demanded my test paper. She shuffled some papers on her desk, avoiding my eyes. "You know, I seem to have misplaced it. Goodness knows what I did with it, but I'll keep looking. I'm sure it'll turn up."

I was naïve but I wasn't buying her story. I told my French teacher and wasn't surprised when soon after the principal called me to his office. I plopped into a chair feeling dejected by my predicament.

"Richard," he said, "I was surprised to hear about your English test grade. You've done so well in the past. I'm going to see if we can have the paper re-read."

"Mrs MacFee says she lost it. I don't think she's going to find it, either." As disheartened as I was, I could tell from his demeanor that the principal seemed to agree that something fishy was going on.

Then he leaned his elbows on his desk, looked me in the eye, and lowered his voice. "Richard, you know that with the war we've had a terrible shortage of teachers. Mrs MacFee is working here filling in for the teachers who are working in the war plants and the armed services. So she has been brought back from retirement."

Then it hit me like a thunderclap – she had proudly told our class that her nephew was in the famous Dover Patrol, a branch of the British Royal Navy that had guarded the all-important Dover Straits during both world wars. The Dover Straits were

England's lifeline and many sailors had died in the first war chasing submarines and keeping the route clear for both attacks and retreats from France.

She spoke with uncommon passion about how her nephew was facing danger and death to protect England from the Axis enemies: the Germans, Japanese ... and the Italians. The way she told us the story of her nephew had made me squirm a little at the time. My family had relatives that still lived in Calabria.

The war had been even closer to our home than that. Through the immigrant grapevine and in the newspapers, those of us on Alice Street knew that Italians in America had to carry special identity cards and couldn't live just anywhere they wanted. In both Canada and America, some had been interned, along with the Japanese and the Germans.

On Alice Street the ethnic groups might complain about each other from time to time, but we shared the common bonds of striving for a better life. It was easy to forget that millions around the world were dying, some of them possibly fighting our uncles and cousins on faraway battlefields.

Mrs MacFee and I ended up with a negotiated settlement, no doubt imposed on her by the principal. She informed me that my paper was in fact lost but she would let me take a makeup test on Shakespeare's *MacBeth*.

She administered an oral exam this time and gave me a 60, a "C". My first failing grade would be removed from the record, she said. "Thank you," I lied. With a great sigh of relief, I graduated out of her clutches into grade twelve.

I had allies in my confrontation with Mrs MacFee, but when I fell in love with the wrong girl, no one could help me with my heartache. I'd met Debbie at a YMCA dance and in time became smitten. She seemed to be as well.

She invited me to tea with her family one Sunday. Her father was an executive with the local factory of a large industrial company headquartered in the States. They lived in a beautiful home and the tea service was all silver and china.

It was clear I was getting the look-over as her mother and father peppered me with questions about who my parents were, and about my brothers and sisters, and what everyone did for a living. Their faces registered shock when I told them I was one of sixteen children, and Catholic. They were Anglicans.

I did my best to hold my own, sufficiently schooled in chemistry to be able to discuss with her father the manufacturing processes in his pipe-making operation. Debbie's mother was gracious and accommodating. All seemed to go well.

Soon after, Debbie asked to meet my parents. We agreed on Sunday dinner. The weather turned out to be miserable – snowy, icy day, slushy – and Alice Street was nearly impassable by car.

Debbie's mother dropped her off without coming inside. There was an awkward introduction, as my parents spoke broken English at best. Then we shared a quiet meal. When dinner was over, Debbie called her mother to come pick her up. The large Hudson came slithering down the street through the ice and snow. Her mother had to fight the steering wheel – this in the days before power steering – to keep the car in a straight line.

When she stopped in front of the house she was breathing heavily from the exertion and her face was grim. My heart sank. I knew from her cold demeanor that it was probably over with Debbie. As she got into the car, her mother was sizing up the neighborhood, scanning with hawkish eyes the house, my family, and me.

Then the car was gone.

Debbie made it official the next day at school. "Richard, my mother says that it would be best if we didn't see each other any more."

She was the first girl I had cared for, and I was crushed, knowing there was no hope of a reconciliation. She had her parents' orders. We never spoke again. All I could do was watch her from afar at school with a mixture of grief, anger, and frustration.

ooooo

True love had eluded me but I found another form of self-expression that led to the most extraordinary experience I ever had with my mother. In the spring of 1948 I signed up on a whim to participate in the school's annual open-invitation track and field contest. I had four athletic brothers who had excelled in track and field and in professional football, so I cockily signed up to compete in every event in the senior division: the mile, 880 yards, 440 yards, and 220 yards.

The three longest races were held after school at a longer track at the Ontario Veterinary College in Guelph, the oldest veterinary school in Canada. The races would be run on three consecutive nights. The final event, the 220, was to be held on our own school grounds on the fourth day.

I worked in the store every night after school, so I had to go to the store after school and then ride my bicycle across town to the college for the race. The first night, for the mile, I arrived to find most of the contestants turned out in matching t-shirts and shorts, sporting new track shoes. All I had was an old pair of scuffed-up running shoes, a sleeveless undershirt, and a pair of old street shorts.

I didn't care about my looks but I worried that my shoes might not hold out. I had never trained for any of these events, so I asked a friend to stand at the inside of the track to tell me how I was doing so I could know whether to speed up or conserve my energy.

At the starting line, I watched and copied what the other runners were doing to prepare to push off. The starter pistol cracked, and I leaped forward like a rabbit flushed from a log.

My pre-race strategy had been to run in the draft of the leader, settle into a steady pace, and then make my move near the end. But I realized as I rounded the first corner that there was no one in front of me. That was confusing because one of the runners in my heat was the current record holder and another was a local hockey star.

I scolded myself for starting off at too brisk a pace. I turned my head to see the rest of the runners and found a star college athlete hot on my heels. I was being drafted, instead of the other way around. I poured on extra speed.

The first quarter-mile mark approached, the spot where my friend was supposed to be standing to shout me his instructions. But he wasn't there. I glanced across the track infield and saw stragglers half a lap behind me. I might be running too fast, but I still had a rival right behind me. I concentrated on keeping up my pace.

At the half-mile mark I turned and my rival was gone. I spotted him lying on the inside of the track, clutching his side and gasping for breath. The next closest runner was a hundred yards back. Going into the fourth and final lap, I felt like a Serengeti gazelle that had outrun a cheetah.

I sprinted all the way to the finish line. It took me a hundred yards to come to a stop. People I didn't know were slapping me on the back. I had run the mile in 5 minutes, 2 seconds, breaking the local record by 29 seconds. I was on cloud nine, until I remembered that I had to get back to the store. I quickly changed and pedaled as fast as I could across town.

The next two days were repeats. I broke the 880 and 440 records, and won the 220 by a split second. I was the senior boys Field Day Champion.

I went across the street from school to a grocery store with a telephone and called to tell my mother the good news. "Dio lo vuole!" she cried.

When I got home, I told her all about the race. "All that running!" she said. "Your feet must be tired." I shrugged.

"Assedetti!" she ordered. I sat down in a chair at the dining table wondering what we she was up to. She bustled into the kitchen and came back a minute later with a basin of warm, soapy water.

She startled me by kneeling and proceeding to untie and pull off my shoes and socks, just as she had many years before when I was a child. Then she pushed the basin close and lifted my feet one by one into the soapy water and washed each thoroughly, telling me all the while how much better this would make them feel.

I was bemused and touched. Although I was an eighteen-year-old man, she seemed determined to perform this ritual. I sat quietly, listening to her talk, as she lovingly washed and dried my feet. Then she stood up, hands on hips, a satisfied smile on her face.

"Grazie, Ma. Grazie! Mi piedi sentino bene." My feet felt great. I kissed her on the cheek and dragged my tired body off to bed.

It would be years before I fully understood that there had been more at work than a mother's nurturing instinct. It had been an expression of her profound love for me and a manifestation in its symbolism of her religious fervor. Like the clumsy hunting expedition with my father, it became one of my most cherished memories.

PART II
UPHILL ALL THE WAY

CHAPTER EIGHT

JACKHAMMERS AND PANCAKES

Inspired by Silvio's example, I began to think about a career in medicine, although I wasn't sure if I had the temperment and I knew it would be a huge financial challenge. I graduated from my final, college prep year of high school in 1948, ready to go to college, but Dominic insisted I'd have to work in the store fulltime for a year to save enough money. So I put my education on hold.

That fall, a chronic pain developed in my right ear. It was diagnosed as mastoiditis, an infection of the bone behind the ear, a condition often caused by an untreated middle ear infection. Years ago it was a leading cause of child mortality. The doctor said I'd need surgery to clean out the infected bone.

When I reported the diagnosis to my family, Dominic's wife, Lola, a registered nurse, questioned whether an operation was necessary. It was a great expense, and she suspected the doctor of exaggerating the risks to increase his business.

Fresh in her memory was the costly operation I had needed a year earlier to repair a hernia I had gotten from lifting heavy sacks and crates in the store. Dominic bore the brunt of the medical expenses, and my productivity suffered for a while as well. Against this backdrop, Lola persuaded me to wait and see about the mastoidectomy. Maybe the problem would clear up on its own. The pain was dull enough that I could stand it, so I waited.

My brother Mike, who was living in Montreal and operated a machine shop, wrote to me in November inviting me to come work for him at a higher salary. Dominic and Lola surprised me when they immediately agreed that it was a good idea. My ear was still troubling me, and they no doubt were relieved that if I did need surgery, they wouldn't get stuck with the bill.

For my part, I was excited to get out from under Dominic's authority and see some of the world. As my father faded, Dominic became a father figure, for better and worse. By contrast, Mike had been my champion when he persuaded Dominic to let me start high school over again, so I could be in the college prep program.

A few days after getting Mike's letter and writing back my acceptance, I rose in the pre-dawn darkness, stuffed my worldly possessions into a duffel bag, tucked $19 in paper currency into my shoe, pulled on my parka and gloves, hiked across town in the cold to the main highway, and stuck out my thumb. It took me all day to cover the 600 kilometres and finally reach the house two cousins shared in Baie-d'Urfe, a small river town about 35 kilometres west of downtown Montreal. To save my money, I had hardly eaten anything and gratefully sat down to the large, hot meal they had prepared.

My brother and cousins owned several businesses and I was shifted from one to another during the next few months, depending on where I was most needed. I worked many days in the family's metal fabrication shop, operating a stamping machine that turned sheet aluminum into struts for television towers. Another relative owned a furniture and appliance store where I sometimes helped out.

By Christmas I had saved up the train fare to go home to Guelph for the holiday. The pain in my ear had worsened and I spent the visit feeling sick, depressed, and fatigued.

I returned to Montreal a few days later, but this time I bunked with another brother and his family in Valois, a Montreal suburb. My brother, Steve, and his wife, Marge, had a small house and three children, but they made a place for me to sleep under the stairway next to the stove where I would be warm.

My misery deepened and I woke a few days later to find my pillow stained with pus and blood. The next morning I opened my eyes to find Steve and Marge standing over me with worried looks. I had been moaning all night, they said. "You need to go to the hospital right away."

I dressed and dragged myself to the station where I caught a train to Montreal Central. From there I walked past McGill University and up the hill to the emergency room at Royal Victoria Hospital. Several doctors examined me, I was x-rayed, and Dr E. A. Stuart, the ear, nose, and throat specialist on duty, sat me down and delivered the news: the infection had eaten away most of the mastoid bone and would soon break through to my brain, in which case I could easily die of meningitis.

He sent me home to tell my family, grab my toothbrush, and come back. I was admitted and prepped for surgery, which took place the next morning. I had a radical mastoidectomy, which meant I lost all hearing in my right ear.

My first awareness when coming out of the anesthesia was the sound of someone wailing loudly nearby, in an unfamiliar language. I reached up and felt the bandage that was wrapped all the way around my head, from jaw to pate.

I gingerly rotated my head enough to see a Rabbi leaning over the man in the bed next to mine, praying loudly and gesticulating. I had spoken briefly to that man the night before and learned he was also having a mastoidectomy.

I couldn't figure out what all the fuss was about at first, and then I noticed that along with the same kind of bandage I had, he also had a patch over one eye and one side of his mouth looked droopy. After the Rabbi and visitors left and the ruckus calmed down, I asked him what was wrong. A facial nerve had been damaged during the operation, which had left him with partial paralysis, including the inability to blink or close one eye. He had to wear a patch to keep the unblinking eye from drying out.

The man's predicament was chilling. "Dio lo vuole," I heard my mother's voice say. I sent up a silent prayer, thanking God for sparing me from such a tragedy. Being half-deaf seemed trivial by comparison.

I was wheeled back into the operating room the next morning to have the packing removed from my ear. The doctor first tried to remove the dressing without anesthesia, but a lot of blood had clotted and when he tugged on the packing, I screamed in pain. So they put me under.

When my condition improved, they sent me home and back to work with a bandage over my ear to catch the seepage of fluids from the surgical site. I also had to regularly redress a small patch on my right thigh where the surgeons had harvested a skin graft to put into my ear canal to close up the wound there.

Being deaf in my right ear took some adjusting. I quickly learned to sit on the right of anyone who was speaking to me.

ooooo

By April I was feeling well enough to be restless. At five cents an hour plus room and board, my family machine-shop job would take me forever to earn what I needed for college and I knew better than to ask Dominic for help. I started reading the classifieds.

The *Montreal Star* had an ad for construction laborers to work at Goose Bay Air Base in Labrador. The jobs started in May and paid 69 cents an hour plus room and board, ten hours a day, six days a week. I recruited a friend, Jack Harcourt, who was in a similar situation to mine, trying to save money for school, and we went down to the Sun Life building in Montreal for an interview.

A large bomber hangar had burned down at Goose Bay and a contractor was hiring a crew of men willing to go out in the boondocks to clear the wreckage and rebuild. We were warned that it was "bull labor" – hard physical work. Jack and I were young and strong, so we both got hired. A month later, we were strapped into an Air Force DC-4 and flown nearly a thousand miles across the vast, empty, lake-laced landscape of northern Quebec and Newfoundland to the end of Maritime Canada: Goose Bay.

The Goose Bay Air Force Base had been built during the Second World War and for a time had been the largest airport in the world. When Jack and I got there, it was between its busiest period during the war and a coming build-up as a major US radar site and bomber base during the Cold War.

The base had been built on a high plateau in a mountainous region so far north that the climate supported only small, stunted cedars. It was cold and damp most of the time, although the summer days were long.

We lived in a barracks with sixty-five other men, who included Eskimos, Labradoreans, Maritimers from New Brunswick, and eastern Canadians. Every morning a big truck would pull up next to the mess hall and we'd all pile in like cattle to be driven off to the hangar site. We worked with jackhammers, picks, and shovels to break up the concrete, haul the debris away, and remove old gas tanks and other ruined equipment. Being taller and stronger, I was assigned to a large jackhammer weighing 110 pounds.

When we got to the rebuilding phase, we moved, by hand, 200-pound slabs of concrete from a ship to a waiting truck on the dock. It turned out to be as advertised – "bull work" – and at the end of each day I ached in every joint and muscle. Working ten hours a day, there was enough time to eat, clean up, and sleep – nothing more. Sundays we enjoyed the supreme luxury of sleeping in.

A saving grace of that desolate place was a library, which I visited every chance I got, reading all the science books I could find. I also read *Babbitt* by Sinclair Lewis.

I took some Italian lessons by correspondence with a classics scholar I knew who had studied at Yale and lived in Guelph. I was eager to improve my Italian for times when I was around my family. I had two cousins, girls, who delighted in mocking me when I tried to speak the Calabrese dialect, which was quite different from the classical Italian of Dante's *Divine Comedy* that I had studied in high school.

Before I left for Goose Bay I had gone to Royal Victoria Hospital to have sulfa crystals squirted in my right ear to hasten the healing. But the graft of thigh skin over the hole in my head continued to drain. Doctors at Goose Bay assured me that it was clear drainage, so there was no infection. They gave me a shot of penicillin every week which stopped the drainage and the last of the pain.

ooooo

With few distractions and our bodies working hard all day, we labourers always looked forward to hearty meals. The cook was an old, hunched-over Russian immigrant named Kuzma Tymoshenko, who chain-smoked and spoke with a thick accent.

Kuzma complained constantly that the construction company was underpaying him. He demanded a raise but they ignored him, which fueled his fury. One day he announced that he was quitting and would leave on the next day's flight out. His superiors insisted that he find a temporary replacement until another full-time cook could be recruited and flown in.

I learned all this because Kuzma came to me and, in his thick Russian accent, announced, "You are only guy can read and write, and you work in grocery store. I teach you to cook. Tomorrow I go and you are new cook."

I protested. "I'm a jackhammer operator. What do I know about cooking?"

"You write what I tell you," he said. "Then you can cook."

The first thing I learned was that I had to make more than a hundred flapjacks every morning. Kuzma showed me how to mix the batter in a big barrel and set it in the fridge overnight. He gave me the rest of my instructions and the next day after I worked with him on breakfast, he said goodbye and flew away, leaving me to figure out the rest.

The stove was enormous, twelve or so feet long. Once I had all the burners turned up and the griddle hot, I dipped a large ladle into the batter and went as fast as I could pouring pancakes. By the time I got to the end of the row, I had to rush back to turn them all over before they burned.

The morning after Kuzma left, the head of the construction company, Mr Brittan, came in for his usual breakfast, smoking a pipe, dressed in a three-piece suit. He walked up to me and, in a heavy Scottish brogue, asked, "What are you doing here, Valeriote?"

I explained that I had been recruited to fill in until a real cook could be found. Curiosity satisfied, he sat at a table and waited for his pancakes.

When I set his plate in front of him, he looked down, scowled, and asked, "What the hell are you doing?"

"What's the matter Mr Brittan?"

"This is maple syrup you've poured on here!"

"Yes sir. It's all I've got, cases of maple syrup."

"You're supposed to be using a ten to one mix!" His tone was indignant. "Nine parts corn syrup for every one part maple syrup. What the hell are you trying to do, serving pure maple syrup?"

"Mr Brittan, pure maple syrup is all I've got."

"This stuff costs a fortune!"

I had worked in the family grocery store long enough to know he was right, and I could only imagine what it cost to ship it to Goose Bay.

"It's all we have. There's no corn syrup to mix it with."

He sighed. "I'll have some sent from Montreal right away. Just go easy on the maple in the meantime."

Another thing I knew from working in the family business was butchering, and it was a second reason Kuzma picked me out to replace him. The company flew in whole sides of beef and my job was to butcher the sides into steaks and roasts. What was left over I made into stew.

The chicken we got was tough, probably from being frozen for a long period of time. We called it seagull meat. I had to boil it for hours and load it with spices.

Eggs were stored in a locker next to the beef. We had plenty of eggs but many of them were so old that when you'd break them open all you'd find was blue-green powder. I had a suspicion that some of them were left over from the war. I spent quite a lot of time sorting through eggs looking for ones that were still liquid.

Because the eggs were so old, the only safe way to serve them was in well-cooked omelets with plenty of salt, pepper, and Tabasco to kill the sulfurous smell. But the food was all free and everyone was working so hard they had big appetites. No one seemed to mind much.

ooooo

Traffic in and out of the base was fairly frequent, with overseas flights between Europe and the US stopping for refueling. The base had just been through a busy period during the Berlin Airlift, when the NATO allies defied a Soviet blockade by flying food and other essentials into the free zone of the former German capital.

It later became clear that the work we laborers were doing in 1950 was, in part, preparation for Goose Bay becoming a major North American Strategic Air Command base, home to enormous, long-range bombers that carried nuclear weapons twenty-four hours a day in the skies of the northern hemisphere throughout the Cold War.

One of the more notable touchdowns occurred one day when our boss, Mr Tremblay, ordered us to shut off the giant compressor driving the jackhammers and move away from the tarmac. The silence was broken by the approach and landing of an enormous four-prop airplane. It taxied over to where we were standing.

The plane, a new Boeing 377 Stratocruiser, rolled to a stop and shut down its engines. Tremblay told us that it was a new luxury liner on its maiden flight from Shannon Airport to Los Angeles.

"And fellows, you'll never guess who's on board so I'll tell you. Bing Crosby!"

There was no bigger recording star in the world at the time, and he was the number one box office draw. We crowded around the stairway and when the door opened, there was Bing Crosby looking dapper and very short, wearing an elegant sports jacket and trimmed Fedora.

He smiled and waved to everyone, then strolled down the stairway and loitered around the tarmac with the other passengers while the plane was refueled. It was all over in under a half-hour and then the plane roared off.

ooooo

During my Goose Bay summer, Jack and I applied to colleges. We both applied for admission to McGill University, as candidates for the science program. I also applied to the University of Western Ontario, which was Silvio's alma mater. I knew McGill was highly competitive, attracting the best students from around the world, so I tried not to get my hopes up. I had a fallback plan, to study geology at a college in Newfoundland.

Both Jack and I were accepted by McGill. Western was eager to have me because of my skill as a track and field competitor.

But I knew I'd have to work nights to pay my way through college, leaving no time for sports. McGill's reputation and prestige were reason enough to choose it over Western. McGill had established a worldwide reputation for scholarship, especially for its medical school. It was a great opportunity and I was determined to make the most of it.

By the end of that summer, I had saved $525, equal in buying power to about $5,000 in 2007. It was a handsome nest egg, although I'd still have to work my way through college.

As a military installation shared with the United States Air Force, Goose Bay had an American-style store for personnel, called a PX. You could buy a lot of basics there at bargain prices. I decided to stock up on socks, sweaters, and other clothing I would need and purchase my first wristwatch.

The PX was across the main runway, on the American side of the base. The runway was a mile long, actively used, and it was forbidden to walk across it. I looked across at the PX, just a couple hundred yards away, and then down the long runway, so long you could hardly see the end of it.

I was too impatient to walk all the way around the runway. I saw no planes and no one around to report me, so I began to quickly stride across the rubber-stained concrete. I was about halfway across when I felt the concrete shudder.

I turned to my right and stared into the silver and glass nose of a four-engine B-29 Superfortress bomber, the same kind that dropped the atomic bombs on Japan. It bearing down on me at full take-off throttle. Its wings seemed to span the entire width of the runway. An enormous, powerful aircraft was about to run me over or cut me to ribbons.

I dropped to the ground a split second before the pilot managed to wrestle the plane into a sharp takeoff. He'd probably seen me long before I saw him. The bomber roared past fifteen feet above my head.

I was stunned, and in a world of trouble. I jumped up and ran like a track star back where I'd come from and straight into some bushes. I hunkered down, expecting any second to hear the rotors of a helicopter come to hunt me down. You could be arrested and thrown in jail for crossing the runaway and I had no intention of getting caught.

But no helicopter showed up. Not even a jeep. I sat in those bushes for hours, until it got dark. Then I slipped back into the barracks doing my best imitation of an amateur cook without a care in the world.

It was a great relief when Jack and I finally flew out of cold, desolate Goose Bay. It was snowing when we took off and sunny and warm when we landed in Montreal two hours later. I was happy to be back in civilization and eager to start school. My first task was to figure out how to pay for it.

CHAPTER NINE

LOVE
WALKS IN

My last year of high school counted for a year toward my bachelor of science requirements, so in the fall of 1950 I entered McGill as a sophomore. As soon as I was able, I went to Guelph to see Dominic about getting help for my expenses.

As usual, he said he had none to offer, and suggested I go to the parish, Sacred Heart, to ask about a student loan. I received $300, to be paid back after graduation. Later, Dominic managed to send me $500. Altogether I was able to raise enough so I wouldn't have to work my first year.

That was fortunate because my McGill studies began not on the main campus in Montreal but on the grounds of a former Royal Canadian Air Force Base at St Jean, Quebec, about fifty kilometres southeast of the city, near the US border. It was known as Dawson College and had been set up five years earlier to accommodate the flood of returning Second World War veterans.

The campus was so far outside the city, and in such a remote area, that the university provided room and board. Even if I had needed to work, there were no jobs close by.

The dorms were clean and tidy, a luxury compared to the rough Goose Bay barracks. The food was excellent, there was plenty of it, and the isolation was conducive to studying. My ear had stopped draining, so I was able to settle in and begin to enjoy my new life as a student of geology, zoology, and so on.

The next year, as a junior taking a premedical course load, I moved onto the Montreal campus. The first half of that year I roomed with another aspiring pre-med student, Zoltan "Zoli" Petrany, who I'd known in high school and at Dawson. Our apartment was on Drummond Street, right up from the Ritz Carlton and close to the student union on Sherbrooke Street.

The evening before classes were to begin, Zoli and I strolled over the gymnasium to check out the "Freshy Hop," an annual social event to kick off the school year. We were tired from moving into our apartment, and after a quick survey of the crowd, we decided to call it a night.

As we were about to leave, a mob of late-comers surged up the stairs blocking our exit. At the foot of the stairs I spotted two girls who were threading their way up through the crowd.

I was feeling good so I nudged Zoli. "See those two girls at the bottom of the stairs? I'll take the short one, you take the tall one." He spotted them and said, "Okay." When the girls got to the landing, we immediately introduced ourselves. The short one was Polly and the tall one was Sue. Both accepted our invitations to dance.

I was smitten from the start, but I had to keep asking her to repeat herself. She was speaking English, but she was from Texas and her accent was barely intelligible. She was lovely to look at, dark-haired with deep dark eyes, as well as intelligent and fun. By the time the dance was over, she seemed as eager as I to continue our conversation, so I walked her to the women's dormitory at Victoria College and we parted agreeing to see each other the next day.

I returned to the apartment feeling the strongest premonition that, in some way or another, this young woman was going to change my life. I slept uneasily, anxious for the next day to start, anxious to see Polly again.

We found each other, more by coincidence than intention. It turned out she was in my psychology class, along with her friend Sue. After that, we became an item. So did Zoli and Sue, so we went overnight from being a couple of young bachelor wingmen to being part of a little family. We did almost all our socializing – football games, dances, and so on – as a foursome.

Polly's father was an American diplomat, an Air Force colonel who had been assigned to the US embassy in Ottawa as senior military attaché to Laurence Steinhardt, President Truman's ambassador to Canada. Her father had worked for Ambassador Steinhardt for years, since the Second World War when Steinhardt, a Jew, had been posted to Turkey. Her father had helped Steinhardt assist in the rescue of some Hungarian Jews from the Bergen-Belsen concentration camp. Steinhardt also helped many eminent intellectuals fleeing Europe find refuge in Turkey.

Only six months before I met Polly, Steinhardt had died in a plane crash in Ontario on a flight to Washington. Polly had practically grown up around the Steinhardts. They were part of her extended family, so the loss was still heavy on her heart. The death of her father's boss also meant her father's career future was up in the air.

Her family history was exotic but also intimidating to a small town immigrant kid. Her parents lived in Rockcliffe Park, the wealthiest neighborhood in Ottawa. I was an impoverished science major with a hard road ahead if I hoped to get into and pay for medical school. My only other experience with love had also been with a daughter of privilege in Guelph, and that had ended with the girl's parents forcing her to dump me.

I was relieved when Polly's father treated me well from the start, complimenting me on my scientific knowledge and language skills. Her mother, however, required convincing. Although she knew Polly and I were going steady, she arranged it so Polly was introduced to a series of smitten cadets and officers from

West Point and Annapolis. Happily, none of them managed to turn her head.

Toward the end of the school year, Polly announced that her father was being reassigned to a base in the States. She would surely be going with her parents.

My stomach flip-flopped. "Where would you go?"

"It could be anywhere," she said, biting her lip. "We've lived in Turkey and in the Philippines. Alaska could be next."

The thought of Polly being so far away was too much to contemplate. I knew I'd lose her if we were separated for a whole year. It was time to act. We were close enough that I felt confident she'd accept my proposal of marriage, but we hadn't discussed it. In those days the social custom required the girl to wait to be asked.

"I'll never see you again if you move away, so let's get married now." We discussed the obvious cons – no money – but there was no question that we each felt meant for the other, so we agreed.

I needed a ring and chose one that cost $100. To pay for it I took some extra work in my brother's metal shop, and sold some odds and ends. I had an extra tube of toothpaste that I sold to another student and a suit that had been given to me by a clothing merchant in Guelph, a Mr Elkins.

From the time I borrowed the $300 from Sacred Heart, I began to keep a list of all the people who helped me with my school expenses. And I wasn't shy about asking, especially around Guelph where my brother Silvio had been a community leader, as well as one of the town doctors.

Instead of a cash loan, Mr Elkins gave me about $500 worth of clothing, perhaps one of the most unusual student loans of many I received. One of the things I got as part of that loan was a teal-colored suit that fetched $20 from a lathe operator I worked with.

I managed to raise the money for the ring in time to propose to Polly at the end of the 1951 school year. She accepted, but worried about how we would survive financially. We were still students. I had one more year of undergraduate school to go, and then, hopefully, medical school. She had two years left to earn her bachelor's of arts.

With the heady optimism of youth, accustomed to doing without and unafraid to ask for help, I said, "I'll figure out a way to borrow enough for both of us to live and go to school. As the proverb says, 'Might as well be hanged for a whole sheep as to be hanged for a lamb.'"

My optimism was borne out when her parents volunteered to pay Polly's expenses for the coming year, a huge help. There was also the question of religion. Polly was Protestant but she became a Catholic prior to our marriage and was confirmed by Cardinal Leger in Montreal.

We were married at St Brigid's Church in Ottawa on 30 August 1951. Only Ambassador Steinhardt's widow attended and noted that I was built much like her husband. She later gave me some of his tailored winter suits, cut from heavy tweeds. I was delighted and felt very stylish. The suits kept me toasty as I trudged up and down the snow and wind-blasted streets of wintertime Montreal. The trade-off was that I sat sweaty and miserable through lectures in classrooms overheated by hissing radiators.

Polly and I settled into a basement apartment in Westmount, the English-speaking part of Montreal, and I concentrated on earning the grades that would get me into medical school. I was a good, conscientious student but I was competing with a lot of other good, conscientious students. There was camaraderie among us, but also the awareness that the odds were long – out of 2,500 applications, the medical school would only accept about 100.

I approached each exam like a general planning a brilliant military campaign. I tried to anticipate the difficult questions and plan how I would answer them. After each exam I went back to my books and checked my answers, trying to forecast my grade. When the final grades were posted, I was shocked to see that my physical chemistry grade was a B. I was certain that I had earned an A and was baffled. I had enjoyed the lectures, the subject matter posed no special problems for me, and I went over the questions again and again, rewriting the exam in my head. Every time I came up with a mark that was 10 points higher and would have earned me an A. My curiosity was intense. That one grade could make the difference. I had to know what I had gotten wrong.

With trepidation, I went to the administration building where a helpful clerk arranged for me to meet with someone from the physical chemistry department to review my actual answer sheets. A young chemistry major led me down to the basement to a section of shelves where the tests were kept, and pulled mine from a box. While I watched, he reviewed the exam questions one by one, page by page, looking for errors.

Page 1 was all right. Page 2, the same. Pages 3, 4, 5, 6 … nothing.

"I'm not seeing anything here that suggests your test was incorrectly graded," he commented. "Everything seems to be checking out."

A wave of despair washed over me. I was stuck with that B. Then, he flipped over the last page of the test and muttered something. Then he turned to me and said, "There's your problem. This question was never graded. You got no points for it. Have a seat over there and give me a few minutes."

My heart was thumping as the minutes ticked by in slow motion. I was positive I had answered the question correctly. Finally, he picked up his red pencil, wrote on the sheet, and showed it to me with a grin. A 10!

"Thank God!" I shouted. "Dio lo vuole!"

I pumped his hand and thanked him with gusto. Then I bounded up the stairs and out into a gorgeous, sunny summer day. All seemed right with the world. Soon after, I got the best news of all: I had been accepted to McGill Medical School.

CHAPTER TEN

FORMALDEHYDE AND FAUX PAS

It was with much hilarity and backslapping that the chosen few of our freshman class met for the first time in the medical school's foyer. We were elated, and we were surprised at some of those who were missing. One was the fellow who'd been president of the Premedical Society, a veteran of Korea, and a strong student.

There were also newcomers who'd done their undergraduate work at universities in other parts of the world. One of my classmates was the nephew of Ethiopian Emperor Haile Selassie, one of the most important political figures in modern Africa.

On a visit to Guelph before medical school began, I visited Dr Harcourt, an elderly physician who had once been a partner with my brother Silvio. He gave me his personal copy of Gray's Anatomy, the same one he had used decades earlier when he studied at Western. I was deeply moved that he would entrust to me such a prized possession.

The first lecture on the first morning of my medical education was delivered by one of McGill's legendary professors, Dr C.P. Martin. He was notable for, among other things, the black band he wore around his head to cover an eye he'd lost to a war wound that also took out a piece of his skull that covered the occipital lobe.

Dr Martin's first lecture was about the bones of the hands, the carpals. I listened attentively as he described the navicular bone and went on to discuss its various articulations, blood supply, and adjacent structures.

I had Dr Harcourt's "Gray's Anatomy" open in front me to the pages about the bones of the hand, but I couldn't seem to find anything called a navicular. I tried to sneak a glance at the other students' books, but that didn't help. I thought maybe I was hearing him wrong, because of my deaf ear. But he kept repeating it until I knew I was hearing him right. Then I thought maybe I was in the wrong section of the book. But I couldn't find navicular in the index.

After a half hour of listening to his lecture, feeling hopelessly lost, I began to panic. Had some terrible mistake been made? If I couldn't understand basic nomenclature, maybe I wasn't cut out for medicine. Maybe I should have gone into geology after all.

By the time the lecture was over, I was an emotional wreck. I approached Dr Martin, and explained my problem. "I don't know what it is, but maybe I'm just not cut out to be a doctor."

He laughed, a response that struck me as odd and even a little off-putting. I was having a major crisis and I saw no humor in it whatsoever.

"Let me see your book." I handed it to him. He chuckled.

"Here's your problem. You're using Gray's Anatomy. You're supposed to be using Cunningham's Anatomy."

"What's the difference. Anatomy is anatomy, right?"

"The terms in Gray's are in Greek. In Cunningham's, they're in Latin. The carpal bone is navicular in Latin, but scaphoid in Greek, even though they both mean boat-shaped. No wonder you couldn't understand the lecture. Read up on it tonight and you'll catch up by tomorrow."

I damn near burst into tears of relief. I wasn't stupid and my hearing was good enough. I went straight to the bookstore and bought my copy of Cunningham's. The next time I went to Guelph, I gave Dr Harcourt his Gray's Anatomy back with thanks.

ooooo

Medicine opened up a whole new world. Instead of dissecting shark and dog bodies, as we had in our undergraduate classes, we would now be working on human cadavers. The classroom was a surreal setting. There were 120 students gathered in a large room with 30 cadavers lying on dissecting tables. The bodies were draped in white sheets soaked in formalin, a mixture of formaldehyde and water, to keep the flesh flexible and prevent rotting. The stinging odor of formaldehyde made my eyes water.

The bodies came to the university from donations, homeless people who had frozen to death, or hobos who had been riding in refrigerated railroad cars and didn't realize until it was too late that they were inhaling carbon monoxide from the compressor units. Every one of those cadavers had stories to tell, but none of us would ever hear them. They were now nameless bodies in service to the healing arts.

When bodies arrived at the school, they were submerged in a tank of formaldehyde in the basement of the anatomy building. A person called a prosector had the job of making sure the cadavers were set up and ready for us students at the start of each class and returning them to storage in between, keeping them covered in white sheets saturated with formalin. It required strength and our prosector looked the part, burly like a longshoreman.

Four students were assigned to each cadaver, and each of us would take rotating roles: one read from the text, one performed the dissection we were studying, two observed and made notes for all. My fellow cadaver-mates were two boys from Bermuda – John Stubbs and William "Bill" Cooke – and another from Montreal, John Ensinck. I was the only one who came from modest roots, but it didn't seem to make any difference to them.

Our cadaver had been a man of between sixty and seventy years old when he died. Like the other cadavers, the formaldehyde had turned his skin yellow and leathery. The first time a medical student works on a cadaver is often a defining moment. It is a test of one's potential for becoming a great doctor, and sometimes students fail that test early on.

One of my classmates was the son of a doctor who had graduated from McGill many years before. He was a good student, conscientious and hardworking, and his whole curriculum had been arranged to get him right where he was, in McGill Medical School. We'd been working on our cadavers for only about an hour that first day when he suddenly blurted, "This isn't how I want to spend the rest of my life!"

In the shocked silence, he pulled off his rubber gloves, removed his smock, and declared that he was quitting medical school, right then and there. It was a stunning turnabout and it was clear he'd made a firm decision. He went around the room saying goodbye to all of us who had shared some or all of his journey, spoke briefly with the anatomy professor, and left the room. Years later I learned that he'd found a satisfying career in public administration.

Dissection for me was not the utterly foreign and bizarre experience it might have been for most, if not all, of my classmates. I had been a butcher, so I was familiar and comfortable with the feel of flesh. Death was no stranger to me, either. I had seen a lot of dead bodies during my altar boy duties and had been close to a number of deaths, like my brother Silvio and young Manny.

My faith, like my mother's, kept me grounded about life's tragedies. Nevertheless, I listened attentively to Dr Martin's opening remarks about our obligation to respect the sanctity and dignity of our subjects. He made it clear that he would tolerate no funny business or practical jokes involving our cadavers. Even the taking of photographs was off limits.

Once we had settled down to work, a somber hush settled over the large room. The only sound was the occasional voice reading from the dissecting manual. Everyone reacts to tension differently and one of my cadaver-mates suggested we could lighten the mood is someone were to tell a joke.

All three turned to me, who liked telling stories, and asked if I knew one. I did and I told it. The punch line caused an explosion of laughter at our table. Every head in the room swung to look at us as Dr Martin stepped smartly toward our table, his one eye with a glint of fire in it.

His gruff Irish brogue echoed off the hard surfaces of the cavernous hall: "What's so funny here?" John Anset turned to Dr Martin and sheepishly uttered words that made my stomach drop.

"Valeriote told a joke, sir." My face burned hot.

"Is that so?" Dr Martin said, his eyebrow arching. "Well, now, perhaps Mr. Valeriote will favor us by going to the front of the class so he can tell it again, and let everyone enjoy his very funny joke."

Dead silence. Terror flooded my soul. I pictured myself being tossed out the front doors of the medical school for inappropriate behavior. My entire career might be ruined by a stupid joke.

Dr Martin nodded toward the lectern, to make it clear at least he wasn't joking. I walked to the front of the class, the condemned man on his way to the gallows, all eyes fixed on me. I grasped the sides of the lectern, took a deep breath, and began, fighting the shakiness in my voice.

"There … There was a young fellow who got his first job, selling suits in a men's clothing store."

I felt like a schoolboy having to stand and make a public confession of some misbehavior. But I figured I'd better try and do a good job of it, anyway. At least I could go out on a high note.

"His first day on the job, the manager explained to the young man that there wasn't much to it since the clothes were already organized by size. A customer could pick whatever he wanted and go straight to the cashier.

"The manager said, 'A true salesman can sell what the store can't get rid of. For instance, see that yellow-checkered suit? It has been out of style for twenty years. It's dusty. Nobody in his right mind would buy it, but a real salesman could sell it.' The manager went back to his tailoring work in the storeroom and left the young man in charge of the selling floor.

"Ten minutes later, the new salesman bursts through the doorway exclaiming, 'I sold it! I sold the yellow-checkered suit.' The manager's jaw hit the floor. Then he noticed that the young man's face was scratched, his tie missing a piece, and his sleeve torn.

"'That guy must have given you a rough time.'

"'No, no,' the salesman said. 'He was no trouble at all. But his seeing-eye dog nearly tore me apart.'"

The entire class of 120 students erupted in raucous laughter. Dr Martin was quaking with laughter. He patted me on the back, and walked away. I never told another joke during dissection.

ooooo

That clumsy first day began our year-long dissection of the human body. We started with the arms and the chest, then moved down to the abdomen, pelvis, and legs. We studied the physical structure of the body down to its smallest detail, understanding where every vein, nerve, and sinew started and ended.

Dissecting is more than just grabbing a scalpel and cutting. It is an art form. You have to move very slowly because if you cut the wrong thing, you can ruin the dissection.

When a body part had been fully disarticulated, it went into a special wooden box. If a student had done a particularly good job of dissecting, Professor Martin or the prosector would take the part from the box and attach small labels to nerves, arteries, muscles, and so forth and then set it aside to be used in the final exam.

The brain was the most challenging, and the last part to be dissected. The first step was to saw through the cranium. It was a tricky thing to do properly and if it was bungled, nothing would look right. So the prosector did this part for us.

The brain fascinated me and I contemplated becoming a neurosurgeon. It is the one organ that has a fourth dimension, its operation, which is in constant fluctuation.

All the regions of the brain had yet to be fully mapped in those days but I found it intriguing that we could already identify that the frontal lobe, the temporal lobe, is connected to emotion and creativity; the front parts of the parietal lobes are for sensory function while the back part is for motor function; and the interior part of the brain that connects to the brain stem controls respiration and circulation.

One of the great privileges of my medical education was the day I got to watch the world-famous neurosurgeon Wilder G. Penfield perform surgery on a tumor-riddled brain. Penfield was a pioneer in the field, inventing a technique called the Montreal procedure that treats severe epilepsy by destroying nerve cells in the brain where the seizures originate. He used electrical probes on patients who were under local anesthesia but still conscious, which allowed him to observe their responses in order to target the responsible areas of the brain.

He created maps of the sensory and motor cortices of the brain that show their connections to the various limbs and organs of the body, maps still used today. During his lifetime Penfield was known as the greatest living Canadian (although he was actually born in Seattle).

ooooo

There were the inevitable mishaps and oddly humorous moments during anatomy that one might expect under such circumstances. One of the students, in violation of the rules, decided to take home an arm he was working on, to study it more closely. When he got off the bus, he forgot the sack with the arm in it. Somehow he retrieved it before he got into trouble.

The annual reunion of medical faculty and students was held at the Ritz Carlton on Sherbrooke Street, and we lowly, first-year students were permitted to attend. It was a big treat, especially for someone like myself for whom such luxuries were unknown.

During the dinner, a man getting out of a cab in front of the hotel was struck by a car, suffering a broken leg and multiple lacerations. The doorman rushed into the ballroom where he assumed there were hundreds of doctors who'd know just what to do.

He grabbed the first person he saw, one of my first year class-mates, and dragged him through the lobby and though the crowd that had gathered around the accident victim on the side-walk. The medical student stood there, rubbing his chin. Finally, the doorman blurted out, "For God's sake, doctor. Don't just stand there. Do something!"

"I can't," the student said apologetically. "We've only studied as far as the arm. We haven't gotten to the leg yet."

ooooo

Polly became pregnant with our first child that year, a joyous development but one that brought with it some complications. She had been working as an assistant secretary for Dr J. Gilbert Turner, chief executive officer of the Royal Victoria Hospital, and we would lose her income when she became a mother.

My obstetrics studies had advanced to the point that I was aware of many of the potential dangers a mother and child faced during delivery. But when Polly announced that "it was time," I took her to the hospital confident of a normal, healthy delivery as she had shown no signs of trouble to that point. So I was surprised when her obstetrician called me in after the delivery to tell me that our daughter, Cathy, had been a footling breech birth, meaning that her foot came out first. I was dismayed because I knew that footling breeches sometimes caused umbilical cord prolapse, an obstetric emergency during labour that threatens the life of the child. It occurs when the water breaks and the umbilical cord falls outside the uterus while the fetus is still inside. The weight of the fetus will often compress the cord, cutting off oxygen and leading to brain damage or stillbirth.

The obstetrician assured me that Polly and Cathy were well with no complications, and in fact they were released in a few days.

About five months later, little Cathy started vomiting and continued to do so all day. I had just studied a condition called pyloric stenosis, when a segment of the small bowel becomes enlarged and obstructs the flow of waste. It is a rare condition, but I became alarmed.

As it turned out I was experiencing a more common malady – medical student disease. That's when medical students start to interpret every symptom they encounter, especially in their own bodies, as evidence of the illnesses they are studying.. Polly called the doctor, got some instructions, and by the next morning Cathy resumed normal feedings.

The experience seemed to substantiate the old medical dictum about playing the odds for various symptoms and taking into account what was most likely. "If you hear hoof beats," the saying goes, "think of horses, not zebras." It was a valuable lesson.

ooooo

Our year of dissection ended with a final exam. All the best specimens, as chosen by Professor Martin and the prosector, were lined
up on a row of tables some fifty feet long. Each disarticulated
organ or body part had numbered tags attached to various tissue
types – arteries, nerves, bone, and so on.

We students were required to start at one end of the row with
a clipboard and write down the name of the tagged parts, what
they did, and so on. No one was permitted to speak, and we did
this one by one. I passed with flying colors. When it was all over,
the cadavers were removed to a cemetery and given proper burial.

CHAPTER ELEVEN

MY MONEY MISSION

By the end of my first year in medicine, the easy sources of funding were gone and I had to look far and wide for money to pay my school bills and support Polly and Cathy. Many weekends I hitchhiked back to Guelph and knocked on every door I could find. After I'd gone through all the relatives and friends, raising a hundred here and a hundred there, I got out a telephone book and looked for familiar names of businesses that might be helpful.

I was on a mission and pride was a luxury I couldn't afford. I walked into many places unannounced, asked to see the owners, and explained my predicament. I was a son of Guelph, the brother of one of Guelph's notable citizens (my late brother Silvio), and I promised to pay back every penny I borrowed.

The majority of these people hardly knew me and were startled at first as I explained my plight – I was half way through medical school and running out of money. There was often a moment of silence while they looked me over. In the end, many agreed.

I discovered through my perseverance that, although my parents barely had two nickels to rub together, my family had a reputation in town for integrity. Many people remarked on it. "Thank God for small mercies," I thought.

Early on in my fundraising I tried to get a loan from the Guelph branch of Dominion Bank. The branch manager was Henry Bassett, known to be wealthy and reputed to have one of the largest collections in the world of British Empire postage stamps.

After I introduced myself, I told him I wanted to apply for a loan. He reached in his desk and pulled out an application. "What is the loan for?"

I explained my situation. He put the application away.

"Young man, I admire your determination," he said. "I do know of you and of your family. I remember reading in the local newspaper about you breaking all those track records in high school. But I can't lend you any of the bank's money because you have no income and your ability to repay the loan is years away. But I feel so certain of your ultimate success, I'll make a loan to you personally." He pulled out a chequebook from his inside pocket and wrote a cheque for $200. Then he made out a promissory note payable in six years, at no interest.

Each success increased my self-confidence and resourcefulness. I took to standing in front of the Dominion Bank, hoping to see someone I could borrow from. On one such occasion, a local contractor named Pagani emerged. I intercepted him and introduced myself, explaining what I was about.

His face lit up. "I know you and your family," he said. "My son went to school with you." He pulled out his wallet and emptied it into my hand. I counted $200 in cash.

He chuckled at the stunned look on my face. "You should have hit me before I went into the bank. I had a lot more."

I suggested we go back inside to make out a promissory note. He dismissed the idea with wave of his hand. "I trust you, and I don't want any interest anyway. You pay me when you can."

On one of my early hitchhiking trips back to Guelph, I was dropped off at the bridge between Île Perrot and Dorion, at the far western approach to Montreal, where the Ottawa River flows into the mighty St Lawrence. It was afternoon, late fall, and as daylight faded from the leaden overcast, an icy breeze blew off the river and a light drizzle began. Traffic was sparse and everyone seemed to be coming off the bridge fast, in a hurry. I began to sink into a funk, feeling sorry for myself, something I rarely indulged. But I was lonely that night and weary of the constant struggle and deprivation.

On Sherbrooke Street, on my regular route to or from school, there was a butcher shop I passed each day that had beautiful, thick steaks and roasts in the window, wrapped in green paper. How often I fantasized about taking a brick and smashing the window to get some of that juicy meat.

So I was in a low mood when a Trans-Canada train came rumbling slowly across the rail bridge that ran parallel to the road I was standing on, headed west toward Toronto. The dining car glided majestically by like an ocean liner, allowing me a clear view of passengers sitting in the golden light, framed by lace curtains, raising laden forks and rosy wine glasses to their mouths, while waiters in starched white shirts and bow ties stepped smartly to meet their every whim. A dream world passed before my eyes in slow motion.

Then the train picked up speed and roared off into the dusky mist. God seemed to be taunting me. I was cold, lonely, and hungry and he had teased me with all I couldn't have: warmth, companionship, and a full belly.

I looked across the highway and spotted a horse, his head jutting toward me over a wire fence that surrounded a barren, muddy pasture. Rain dripped off his withers. He was staring at me, as if to say, "Brother, I know just how you feel!"

I had never communicated with an animal before and have never had an experience like that one since. I felt a powerful bond with that beast as he stood there so still – hooves mired in mud, coat soaking wet – exchanging a long, sad, knowing glance with me in the dispiriting place we found ourselves sharing.

We watched each other like that for almost two hours, interrupted by my stepping out with a raised thumb whenever a potential ride approached. His ears would perk up and he'd turn his head and look down the road with me, as if he were also waiting for someone to come. His hopes were more modest, I thought – a child returning from school with a treat of an apple or a carrot. But I knew exactly how he felt.

A car finally pulled over. I grabbed the door-handle like a lifeline. Just before I got in, I looked across the roof at the horse, who seemed to be watching me with mournful eyes. I waved to him, and scrambled into the warmth of the car.

As I settled in, I said a silent prayer for the horse, that God would send him what he wanted. Those two hours come back to me often, and each time I hope God was as good to that horse as He has been to me.

ooooo

I always presented my loan requests as business deals – I would repay with interest, usually a bit higher than the bank paid. I learned to accept rejection gracefully. No one owed me a hand up, but that didn't stop me from trying to find one. People who turned me down were almost always pleasant about it, but I had a few experiences that were a challenge to my spirits.

A friend who helped me suggested that I also approach his father, who was a successful businessman worth several million dollars. I'd spent a lot of time with the man's son, so when I showed up at his office, he knew who I was and made time to see me.

I presented my case. He immediately picked up a pencil and pad and asked me how much I would need to finish my education. I estimated it at about $5,000. We chatted about the cost of tuition, rent, and all of that. It seemed clear that he was leaning toward helping me. My spirits soared.

Finally, he said, "Richard, how can I be guaranteed that you would repay this loan?"

I proposed to buy an insurance policy for $5,000, naming him as the beneficiary.

"That's fine if you die. But what if you become ill, or a drunkard, and can't repay the loan?"

I was so startled by this remark I couldn't think of a thing to say.

He tapped his pencil on the desk and continued, "You know, we had a fire at the psychiatric institute, and there was no insurance. So I had to pay for the damage myself. If that isn't bad enough, I had to buy my daughter a house. Now I've got to send a deposit to Florida for my vacation there this winter. All of this has depleted my cash, so I'm afraid that I can't help you."

I felt as if someone had started to pat me on the back but instead punched me in the gut. I thanked him for his time and left, drawing on all my emotional willpower to remain optimistic.

There were a couple of other cases that were especially jarring. My high school principal, Fred Hamilton, told me an alumnus of the high school had offered to lend money to a deserving student. Hamilton gave me the man's address and I walked across town to his estate-sized home in Guelph's best neighborhood.

He answered the doorbell. I stated my business and he invited me in. I followed him to the parlor and we both sat down.

"Tell me about yourself," he said.

"My name is Richard Valeriote. I'm a native of Guelph and a graduate of Sacred Heart, and now I'm a student at McGill Medical School."

He stroked his chin and his brow creased. "Valeriote," he said. "You're Italian, and Catholic, aren't you?"

"Yes, but ..."

"Well, I'm afraid I don't have any money for you."

A wave of adrenaline entered my system. My chest tightened. I made a clumsy, hasty retreat.

I walked home in a stupor of disbelief. I had been there, but I couldn't believe it actually happened.

Mr Hamilton fumed and apologized when I told him. "I can't believe he said that to you. If I'd known ..."

Next he sent me to see an alumnus in Hespeler, about nine miles from Guelph. "He has a desire to lend money to deserving students."

Again I reeled off my pitch only to be told that he had already lent the money he'd set aside for students.

Poor Mr Hamilton was humiliated and apoplectic. "I am so upset by all this that I'm going to lend you money myself." He wrote a check for $200 and I signed a promissory note at 5 percent.

That same trip I went to see Mr Pagani, from whom I had borrowed money in front of the bank. He loaned me another $300 in cash and once again refused to take a promissory note.

Someone had told me that Louis Ferraro, who lived down the street from my parents at 51 Alice, might be able to help me. I had to leave for Montreal early the next morning to get home before dark. It was late, but I couldn't leave any stones unturned. I knocked on his door at 11 o'clock at night.

Louis's father answered and let me in. He said Louis was asleep in his room at the top of the stairs. I was so full of determination that I walked right up the stairs and into Louis' bedroom, waking him from a deep sleep.

He sat up, blinking, startled, and then he stared at me in disbelief. "Louis, I'm sorry to wake you up like this, but I'm in my last year at McGill and I'm broke. Can you lend me some money, anything?"

He sighed, left his bed, and went to a chest and pulled open a drawer. He reached under some socks, and pulled out a wad of bills. He counted it. "Here's a hundred dollars. Pay me back when you can." Then he yawned and crawled back into bed.

By the time I graduated from medical school, I had a list of more than forty such loans, all of which I eventually repaid or were forgiven. For example, I was visiting my parents on my way to my internship in Flint, Michigan, when there was a knock on the door. It was Mr Bassett from the bank.

"Congratulations!" he said. "I read in the newspaper that you graduated from McGill and I wanted to give you a present." He handed me the promissory note for $200, torn in half. I nearly hugged him with gratitude, not for the $200 but for the trust he had placed in me.

In one instance, I repaid a life insurance brokerage, sending the money by mail. It had been so many years since I borrowed it that they had forgotten about the loan. They were so impressed by my honesty that an employee tipped off the newspaper, which published a short item.

ooooo

The summer between my first and second years of medical school, I got a job with Northern Electric, a subsidiary of Bell Telephone, on a crew that was erecting transmission towers. I worked twelve hour days, six days a week, resting only on Sundays.

One day, before work, I responded to an urgent blood drive by the Red Cross at the McGill student union. I had run out of the apartment that morning without breakfast. I gave the blood and then went on to work.

I was holding on to a long aluminum wire connected to the tower we were putting up when the tower became unsteady and the three of us had to struggle to keep it from swaying while we anchored it to the concrete footing.

It was a warm day and I began to sweat heavily. Suddenly I felt faint. I cried out to my fellow workers that I thought I was going to pass out. Someone relieved me as the tower swayed back and forth. I lay down while someone ran to fetch me a doughnut and a cup of coffee. I recovered and figured I had suffered from low blood sugar.

But as I started my second year, I grew more and more tired and weak. I had lost weight over the summer and figured it was just a seasonal thing. But that fall I continued to lose weight.

Halfway through the year, I began to have chills and fevers with night sweats and a need to urinate frequently. I saw a doctor at the University Medical Clinic, who diagnosed a urinary tract infection and prescribed sulfa drugs. The sulfa triggered a rash. I went back to the doctor, who said I seemed to be improving and discontinued the medication. But the chills and fever and weight loss continued. I returned to the clinic for more tests.

I was still making the trips home searching for money, but by this time I had met a trucker who drove the Montreal-Toronto route regularly and offered to give me a ride any time I needed it. This was a tremendous improvement over hitching all the way.

One cold winter night he dropped me off in Toronto and I continued hitchhiking down the Queen Elizabeth highway to Hamilton to Highway 6, which turned off north to Guelph. I stood at this junction for some time with cars whizzing past my outstretched thumb. It began raining and then the rain turned to sleet. My clothes became soaked and then began to harden as the moisture turned to ice.

It was pitch dark, so motorists couldn't see me until they were just about on top of me. Ice was forming on the road. A large truck came barreling out of the darkness and the driver must have been startled to see me so close to the road because he swerved, sending an avalanche of water cascading off the tarpaulin covering his load and all over me.

I had never been so cold and miserable. I knew that if I didn't find shelter soon, I was in danger of hypothermia. There was a café about three miles up the road so I struck out walking. It was all uphill, a long grade, and no one stopped to pick me up. I trudged on thinking all the while that if I stopped, I would probably die of exposure. When I reached the café I went straight to a seat nearest a steam radiator. I ordered a cup of coffee. Ice began to fall off my clothes, puddling on the floor.

When I finally warmed up, I placed a collect call to Dominic in Guelph, about twenty-six miles away. "You picked the worst night of the year," he said. "The highway is all glare ice. I'll put the chains on but it'll take a while to get there."

He finally made it. On the ride home I sat in the front seat rubbing my hands in the warm air from the heater, but I still felt like an icicle. When I arrived home at 2 o'clock in the morning, my parents were waiting up with hot coffee and a plate of spaghetti. I telephoned Polly to let her know I had made it and climbed into bed shivering with chills and achy with fever.

When I got back to Montreal, I went to see the doctor again because I couldn't seem to shake whatever it was that was making me feel so low. But he told me I probably had a case of "med student's disease." I gave a urine and blood sample and dragged my skinny, weak carcass off to school, wondering if it was really possible to psychosomatically lose so much weight and feel so lousy.

A short while later, near the end of that second year, I was walking across the campus to the library to study for my final exams when one of the lab technicians in bacteriology spotted me and approached with a smile on her face.

"Aren't you glad that we finally found out what's the matter with you?"

"What do you mean? What's the matter with me?"

"Don't you know? All the guinea pigs died. You have tuberculosis."

My head began to spin. I thought I might pass out from the shock. The girl's face took on a look of utter horror and she began to cry. "Oh, this is awful! I had no idea you didn't know! I'm so sorry."

I stumbled wordlessly away, in a zombie-like daze. One week from final exams and I've got a devastating diagnosis that makes no sense. I had chills, fever, and weight loss, but none of the coughing associated with tuberculosis.

I went straight to the Dean's office, and he immediately ushered me in and closed the door. He'd already heard that I'd received the bad news in a bad way.

"Richard, I'm so sorry you had to learn your diagnosis like that. We had planned to tell you next week, after you finished your finals. We didn't want you to worry. You have tuberculosis of the kidney. It's infectious only under the most extraordinary circumstances, so you needn't worry about that. But you'll require a year of cure in a sanitarium, until you're well enough to resume your studies."

I was blind-sided and mystified. I knew from my studies that only about ten percent of people infected with *mycobacterium tuberculosis* ever develop tuberculosis disease. Many of those who do suffer TB do so in the first few years following infection, but the bacillus can lie dormant in the body for decades.

Now I learned that people who get TB in the kidneys are often big husky laborers who have been able to resist it in the lung, which is what must have happened to me. I knocked it out of my lungs but it found a new home, spread through the blood. This is called miliary tuberculosis and it is the type that produces fever, weakness, loss of appetite, and weight loss.

My strenuous schedule, the long trips hitchhiking in all sorts of weather, the stress, and poor diet had all combined to weaken my immune system. But where had I been infected? That remained a mystery to me for a few years, until I attended a class reunion and learned that the boy I'd sat right behind, a Japanese-Canadian who had a persistent cough, had ended up in a sanitarium with tuberculosis of the lungs, the most transmittable form. Sam's family had been sent from British Columbia to

Guelph for internment during World War II. But internment in Canada was not as strict as in the States, and Sam was allowed to go to our school.

To my right that year sat Annabelle Peffic and to my left was Jack Howard. The three of us compared notes and discovered that Annabelle had developed a stubborn cough that year, I had the shakes and chills, and Jack's knee became painfully swollen for no apparent reason.

Annabelle, Jack, and I all contracted TB at the same time. It ususally enters through the lungs. Most people can fight it off and never have a problem. In some people, the body throws it out of the lungs but it migrates to some other part of the body. (TB can affect almost any tissue.) Annabelle had it in the lung, Jack had it in his kneecap, and I had it had it in my kidney.

At the time all I knew was that this was a terrible turn of events, all the way around. I would be cooped up in a TB sanitarium for a year, I couldn't work, I had to interrupt my studies, Polly and Cathy would have to go live with family – it turned our lives upside down.

"I suppose you and Cathy ought to go stay with your folks in the States," I told Polly. "My mother would take you in to her house in Guelph in a heartbeat. But that's asking a lot of you, considering the language and culture gap. And my father's no picnic in his own way."

"No, no. I want to stay near you, so we can visit. Besides, I love your parents and it'll give them a chance to get to know their granddaughter. And Cathy can get to know some of her aunts and uncles. We'll make the best of it."

Relieved to have that question resolved, I did my best to pretend my life wasn't in chaos long enough to study well and pass my exams, which I did. We sublet our apartment and went home to Guelph to break the news to my parents.

"Dio lo vuole!" my mother shrugged, arms raised. "This, too, will pass. Before you know it, you'll be back at school."

CHAPTER TWELVE
A YEAR IN "THE SAN"

The Freeport Sanitarium in Kitchener, known as "The San," had been built in 1915 as a military rehabilitation hospital for wounded World War I veterans. It sat on fifteen pristine acres of farm property on the banks of the Grand River. It was in a sylvan, serene, resort-like setting – a great place to be sick.

Like many such facilities, it was surrounded by pine trees because it was thought that something in the trees, some chemical, was good for you. This was never established, but I think the isolation and calm were important. It was also considered healthy to sit in the sun, which is why sanitariums always had south-facing porches and balconies where one could sit and absorb the warmth.

Because it was a hospital filled with people who might be infectious and I was in a depleted state, I started out in a private room, being treated for my fever and chills. I couldn't mingle with the rest of the patients until I'd gotten past those systems.

Life in The San was a sudden, disorienting change at first. I had been very active and had to accept that I was going to be there for the next year walking around in hospital gowns, being pumped full of antibiotics, eating my way back to health, and resting. But I soon settled in and took advantage of the chance to catch up on my reading for the next school year, as well as reading just for pleasure.

The hardest part of being in The San was the separation from Polly and Cathy. But they visited often, and it was clear that mother-in-law and daughter-in-law were getting along well. My mother, who had given birth to sixteen children, loved being a grandma.

When I was healthy enough, I was moved into a shared room with a veterinarian who had tuberculosis of the lung. He was quiet and reticent, a few years older than I. As if he didn't have enough trouble, he managed to contract measles as well. I'd already had measles, so I didn't have to change rooms, but I wished I had when his fever spiked and he started to thrash about from the delirium. They had to tie him down to his bed to keep him from injuring himself. He talked all night, mumbling about aquarium fish. He got so bad they were ready to send him to a regular hospital when the fever finally broke and he began to recover.

I met people from all walks of life in The San. To prevent us from re-infecting each other, each patient had their own gowns with their nametags on the inside. Laundry was boiled in disinfectant soap. We ate meals delivered to us in our rooms instead of in a dining hall. Temperatures were taken daily, blood work and x-rays were done on a regular basis.

The San had an intercom system with speakers in each room, over which we learned about upcoming events and other announcements. It was also used to entertain and I was recruited at one point to host a "broadcast" modeled after a popular radio program at the time called "Twenty Questions." A panel of six contestants had to try to identify an object by asking questions, usually beginning with, "Animal, mineral, or vegetable?"

One of the regular panelists was a young lady from Kitchener named Laurie Hawkes. She was married and the mother of three small children who frequently visited her. She was being treated for tuberculosis of the lung. In addition to antibiotics, food, and rest, she periodically received a procedure which caused an intentional pneumothorax, or collapsed lung.

A needle was inserted into the pleural space between the lung and the chest and air was pumped in which caused one of her lungs to compress by an inch or two. This helped give her lung a chance to rest, and it took a couple of weeks for the lung to fully reinflate.

One day at the end of my Twenty Questions broadcast, she announced that she was about to have her last pneumothorax procedure after which she would be discharged. It always was a cause for celebration and optimism when one of us had regained our weight, been healed, and could go back to our families and lives.

On the morning of Laurie's discharge, we all said our cheery goodbyes as she went downstairs for her last pneumothorax. Her husband and children were waiting in the lobby to take her home.

But this otherwise ordinary procedure that she had experienced so many times before went horribly wrong. Somehow the needle struck her arterial system instead of the pleural cavity and a massive air embolism was pumped into her bloodstream. She died instantly.

The poor doctor was practically suicidal. The procedure called for inserting the needle into the chest cavity and then pulling back to make sure there was no blood. He had done it exactly the same way he always had. He'd never had a problem. He'd never lost a patient that way. But this time was different, and the tragedy was overwhelming. This poor young woman was about to go home after all the heroic efforts to make her well, about to make her victorious exit from The San where she was widely liked and admired. An instant later, her children were motherless and her husband a widower.

As the news spread to the upper floors, the whole building sank into a mournful silence. Everyone retreated to their rooms to lie down and contemplate life's cruel twists of fate. "Dio lo vuole," I thought. But why?

ooooo

Being a medical student can sometimes give you confidence you haven't earned, and that misplaced confidence got me into some painful trouble once. I'd been sent to a nearby hospital in Kitchener to have some special x-rays of my kidneys. X-raying kidneys begins with injecting a dye into one arm. The dye flows through your system until it gets to the kidneys. The x-ray picks up the dye and gives the doctor an image of the exterior of the kidneys.

Following this the doctors needed to see the interior of the kidneys, a procedure requiring a spinal anesthetic to numb the lower half of my body and a urinary catheter to collect samples from each kidney. It was a miserable experience.

I came out of the fog of anesthesia to find a group of nurses chattering away, removing all the things that were attached to my privates. After they'd finished and left, and sensation returned to my legs, I sat up. I was feeling well enough that I decided to get dressed and go downtown to a bookstore to see if I could find something to read.

I knew the nurses would probably make a fuss about my leaving, so I sneaked down the back stairway, caught a bus downtown, went to the bookstore, bought a book, and headed back. But on the way I started to develop a headache that got worse and worse until, by the time I got back to my room, I was in agony.

I called the nurse. "I've got this blinding headache, and I can't stand it."

She called the doctor and while we waited she asked if I had been standing up.

"Yeah," I said, not daring to mention that I'd gone on an adventure downtown.

"You aren't supposed to do that! You're supposed to stay lying down."

That's when I learned that, following a spinal puncture, a bit of spinal fluid can leak out of the hole created by the needle.

The spinal fluid protects the brain and if you lose even a half-ounce of fluid, the brain settles onto the optic nerve, causing a blinding headache that pounds like a sledgehammer.

For the next few days, I had to stay in bed, face down, feet elevated, until my spinal fluid could build back up to normal levels.

ooooo

One of the great frustrations of my year in The San was losing a year of medical school. I received a few letters from classmates now and then, which made me feel good but also made me wistful to be back in the saddle.

One day a letter came from McGill that touched my heart.. I had expected a small refund from the bookstore but was startled to see that the cheque enclosed was for $800 and to read that the money had been collected by my classmates. They had solicited items from businesses in Montreal and then auctioned them off at the student union. The $800 was the profit. I was deeply moved by the gesture, and the money took a great load from my mind. I turned it over to Polly to manage.

The year passed much more quickly than I expected. The chills and fever cleared up, and the day before school started, Polly and I were blessed with the healthy birth of our second child, Susan. We moved back into our apartment in Montreal, and I resumed my education.

My first day I discovered that, although I was healthy, I was not yet strong. Walking up the hill to school I became so weak and dizzy that I had to sit down on a curb for fear I'd keel over in the street. I recovered and paced myself the rest of the way to my first class, pathology. I walked into the hall and sat down with my new classmates, none of whom I recognized. I felt like I was starting over again with a new group of people.

The class was conducted in an amphitheatre by Dean Duff, who was down in the pit with some specimens on a large table.

He looked up and around at us students and when he looked at me he called out my name.

"Valeriote. Will you please come down here."

I walked down the steps into the pit and took my place next to Duff. In front of us were specimens of human brains. Duff pointed to a small pickled brain and asked, "What is this?"

I had to stifle a nervous chuckle. "It is a brain, sir."

"Good," he said. "What else can you tell me about this brain?"

I had been away from school for a year but the Socratic routine felt familiar right off the bat.

"It looks rather small. So it must have been a child."

"You are absolutely right. What else do you notice about the brain?"

It looked diseased. "It's covered with some sort of material. The exterior isn't clean."

Duff nodded. "Why do you think that is? What do you think that covering is?"

"The meninges which cover the brain seems to be affected."

"How did the meninges get in that state?"

This colloquy struck me as odd, and I couldn't figure out why I'd been plucked out of 120 students to participate in it.

"Probably from some kind of infection."

"What kind of infection would produce this type of pattern to the meninges?"

"A granulomas infection might do it."

"What likely granulomas infection would you think that would be?"

Then it hit me and I turned and smiled at Duff. "Tubercular meningitis." He had chosen me because the child whose brain we were looking at had died of the disease I had just overcome: tuberculosis meningitis.

ooooo

My last year of medical school passed quickly. We had graduated from specimens to treating patients with real diseases, which is why I wanted to become a doctor in the first place. A great deal of attention was paid to making accurate diagnoses, a focus I would later learn was one of McGill's strengths.

Although I had raised most of the money I needed to get through school, I was a bit short near the end. But after years of struggling, what we needed suddenly arrived out of nowhere. One morning an administration official from McGill knocked on our apartment door and handed me an envelope. It contained a cheque for $400 from a scholarship fund underwritten by John W. McConnell, a wealthy businessman who owned the *Montreal Star* and had been a benefactor of McGill for many years. One of my guardian angels was Rev. Clifford Knowles, McGill's chaplain and an official in the Student Aid Office. He had made the grant possible, and once again I felt extremely lucky to be trusted by so many.

It wasn't long after, on a wintry Sunday morning at St Patrick's Church, that our priest spoke of the grinding poverty of many people living in the South Pacific. The church was raising money to help them.

"No matter how bad off you think you are," he preached, "there are people in this world who are much worse off. We have a moral obligation to help them. Give and it shall be returned to you one hundred fold."

I nudged Polly and whispered, "How much should we give?"

She grimaced. "Are you kidding? We only have $100 to our name."

I wrote a check for $4.00 and put it in the collection basket.

The next morning the apartment doorbell rang. It was another official from McGill, with another envelope. This one contained another cheque made out to me for $400.

"What is this one for?"

The fellow explained that a child had drowned some years ago in the water-filled excavation at a construction site for a new hospital. The parents had set up an annual scholarship in the child's name to be given to a worthy medical school student. Reverend Knowles had helped me again.

I reminded Polly that I had given $4.00 we couldn't afford the day before and it had paid us back a hundred fold in twenty-four hours.

She laughed. "Then you should have given $10.00."

The week before final exams I was feeling so confident about my future that I agreed to join a friend who wanted to go trout fishing in the Laurentian Mountains north of Montreal. Joe Martin had spotted an article in the newspaper about it and we decided we would play hooky from our classes that day to try our luck.

The trout were biting, apparently easy prey to a lure we were using called a Super Duper. It simulated the wiggling of a fingerling and worked like a charm. But on one of his casts, Joe managed to hook himself in the forehead, just above his nose. We had no pliers or wire cutters to remove it, so I removed the line and Joe continued to fish with the hook imbedded in his head, assuring me that, although it looked Frankensteinian, it didn't hurt.

Soon after we had caught our limit, a fellow fisherman came by carrying a notebook. "I'm a sports reporter for the *Montreal Star*," he explained. "Looks like you're having good luck here." We proudly showed him our fish and gave him our names for his article. "That's 'Valeriote' pronounced like 'lariat'," I said.

Joe said his forehead had finally started to throb and, since we'd caught our limit, we packed up and headed to town. First stop: Royal Victoria Hospital emergency room, where a doctor removed the barb and gave Joe a tetanus booster shot.

The next day, in the first class of the morning, the professor wryly announced, his corners pinched in a suppressed grin, "It must be nice to be able to go fishing the week before exams. Clearly you all know the course material so well you feel confident of passing. I wonder why I even bother to get out of bed."

Joe and I surreptitiously exchanged a beet-red glance, but the professor didn't give us away. After class we huddled in a corner and compared notes. How the heck did the professor know we had been fishing? Did he have a friend in the emergency room? Did one of us tell someone who had a reason to embarrass us?

The same thing happened in the next class, and the next one. By then, other students were turning and grinning at Joe and me. Finally one of them flopped in front of me the *Montreal Star*, to a page with the headline, "Hot Trout Fishing at St. Agathe."

The first line of the story was, "Two McGill students, Richard Valeriote and Joseph Martin, both caught their limits of trout yesterday." One of the professors had handed copies out to all our teachers, who had conspired with each other to have some fun at our expense.

No harm was done and the incident passed with everything but our dignity intact. Both Joe and I mastered our final exams and graduation soon followed, the most exciting moment in my academic career, made all the more satisfying to be sharing it with Polly, my parents, Dominic, and Polly's folks.

After the outdoor ceremony, we all went to dinner at one of the swankier seafood restaurants, Desjardins on MacKay Street, and Polly's parents treated us to lobster dinners. No culture or language gap could diminish the good mood, which in Dominic's case was greatly increased by relief that I was done needing and borrowing money.

Like an ant trying to climb a set of stairs, I had fallen many times but kept at it until I finally reached the top step. How I wished Silvio had lived to share the experience!

PART III
DR VALERIOTE

CHAPTER THIRTEEN

MY YEAR
BEFORE THE MAST

As a graduate of a world-class medical school at a time of a shortage of doctors, my options seemed limitless. The next step was my internship and I could have applied to Royal Victoria Hospital or Montreal General, both prestigious assignments I was qualified for. But these positions paid an honorarium of only $25 a month. I had a wife, two children, and a mountain of student loans. My days of hitchhiking to raise money were over.

One of the opportunities that two of my classmates were considering was in Flint, Michigan. I made a visit and met with the sisters and medical staff at St Joseph Hospital there. I liked what I saw, and I especially liked the idea of earning a living wage. The pay was $200 a month plus an apartment and the hospital would provide food when I was on duty. Polly, the kids, and I would live in nearly new housing right across the street from the hospital. It seemed like an ideal fit.

I bought a used Ford station wagon with $400 I had saved up, borrowed a pickup truck from a friend in Guelph, and moved our family and possessions from Montreal to Flint, where my first day on the job was 1 July 1957. My two McGill classmates were there as well.

My commute was a two-minute walk which meant I could go home anytime I had a break during the day. Polly was pregnant with our third child, Richard, who was born healthy as a horse in September 1957. Because the medical staff lived together in hospital housing, we had a ready-made community of other young doctors whose wives were raising families. While I was off working the long hours, Polly had access to shared resources with other mothers, as well as social events, card parties, and the like. And if she needed me, she could practically holler out the window.

At work I made sure to take full advantage of the free meals. What a guilty pleasure that was after all those years of scrimping and cutting corners. I would never again fantasize about breaking into a butcher shop.

Taking care of people gave me such energy and satisfaction that I found myself silently thanking God for the opportunity. Doctoring had turned out to be all I hoped and then some. I rotated through all the services; medicine, surgery, obstetrics, pediatrics, and my favorite – the emergency room. Ambulances delivered a steady supply of new patients, each one a problem or puzzle to solve. I was in charge of sixteen cubicles, and they were often full of patients needing attention.

St Joseph's got more than its share of trauma cases because it was the nearest emergency room to a major highway that was notorious as a meat grinder. It was the main north-south vacation route between Detroit and Michigan's great outdoors and Upper Peninsula. People drove at break-neck speeds, and we saw quite a few mangled wreck victims.

We also saw a large number of industrial injuries. Flint was a major manufacturing center at the peak of its prosperity. It was the birthplace of Buick and its successor, General Motors, which operated several sprawling plants and office complexes employing more than 80,000 people.

I loved working the emergency room. The adrenaline high was exhilarating, and it was never dull.

One of the things my McGill classmates and I noticed about our education was that the interns from other medical schools seemed to know exactly how to do such basic things as starting an IV or doing a spinal tap. We had never been taught how to do any of that. Our training had been geared toward studying diseases, pathology, bedside diagnosis, treatment, and so on. The prosaic procedures, taking blood and ivs, were performed by technicians, nurses, phlebotomists, and so on.

At McGill, a major teaching university, we had been exposed to a high volume of real cases at the many hospitals in the Montreal area. We McGill medical students had seen so many cases of all the common and many uncommon diseases that we were able to recognize them quickly. We even spent time in an enormous psychiatric hospital and had learned how to identify psychotic behavior and distinguish it from reaction to a medical condition or medication.

So while the other interns had more competence with needles, they were less experienced and confident than we were at figuring out what was wrong with patients and what to do for them. This skill would serve me well in all of my medical career.

One of the stranger cases I handled involved a man who arrived dead. I sent him to the hospital morgue and thought no more of it. But later that day, after my shift had ended, a well-dressed man knocked on our apartment door and asked if I was Dr Valeriote.

I invited him to step inside. He quickly got to the heart of the matter. "This morning you saw Mr McKerring and pronounced him dead in the emergency room."

"Yes, I did."

"Well, he was a car dealer and I'm with the bank that was foreclosing on his business. Regrettably, it seems the shock was too much for Mr McKerring. Either way, we now own a parking lot full of brand new automobiles but we aren't in the car business and need to get rid of them. We would like you to buy one."

I chuckled. "You must be kidding. I'm an intern. You see that I've got young children and a wife to support, plus a pile of school loans to repay. I haven't a dime to spare. I'm sorry."

He raised his hand and said, "Wait, let me explain. We know

you're an intern, but you'll be going into practice soon enough. So we're prepared to let you have the car without making any payments for the first year. We'll hold the title as collateral and in a year you can start making the payments."

Once again, good fortune had arrived on our doorstep at precisely the right moment. The station wagon I'd bought used in Detroit eight months earlier had started making noise in the rear axle and the mechanic had diagnosed a worn-out universal joint that would cost $80 to fix.

"If this is a legitimate offer," I told the man from the bank, "I'll take the biggest car you've got." He assured me it was, so I pulled on my coat and left with him, returning an hour or so later with a brand new, 1957 Ford Country Squire station wagon. It was a blue beauty, with sweeping chrome details on the sides and heavy chrome bumpers. The sticker price was over $3,000.

The next day when the other interns who lived in the adjoining apartments got an eyeful of our new wheels, their jaws dropped and they demanded to know how I was able to swing it. I explained the circumstances, suggesting that "someone upstairs seems to be looking out for us."

ooooo

There were other people looking out for us upstairs, only a few floors up. Principal among them was Sister Digna, the administrator who ran the hospital. St Joseph's had been started in the 1920s by the Sisters of St Joseph. It was first housed in a small convent. By the time I showed up, the hospital had moved and grown to five floors, several wings, more than 400 beds, and 80 bassinets. And it was bulging at the seams.

Sister Digna had the heart of an angel, I'm sure, but she had the brains of a CEO. She would come through the emergency room from time to time, and more than once she would find me stitching up a wound and whisper to me, "Remember, we get paid a dollar a stitch," and wink. So I'd add a stitch or two to keep her happy and the hospital afloat. The prevailing attitude seemed to be that it was all being paid for by the United Auto Workers health insurance, since most of our patients were union members.

She'd also offer to send someone to fetch us a sandwich if we were hungry, a gesture that I thought generous at first until the other doctors clued me in: she wanted us patching people up and keeping the billing department busy, not lollygagging in the doctor's lounge.

One of the more colourful people I worked with there was an older surgeon, Dr Steinman, who had served in the military in a field hospital during World War II. He was chief of surgery and when I wasn't paying close enough attention or not pulling a wound open wide enough so he could see to work, he'd scold me by saying, "Dear, sweet Jesus, Valeriote!"

Perhaps because of his experience, the other doctors referred many of their most hopeless cases to Steinman. These were often patients with multiple complications, including chronic alcoholism and advanced diabetes. As a result, his operating room mortality rate was quite high. One day, during a mortality and morbidity review with the medical staff, Steinman was asked to explain why he'd lost so many patients. This was a moment of high drama and he handled it masterfully.

He stood and said, "I see all you looking smug and wondering how I'm going to talk my way out of this. Well, let's review the record." Then he proceeded to identify every doctor in the room who had referred to him their worst, most hopeless cases, ticking off the inventory of medical horrors they had expected him to overcome. "You guys wouldn't touch these people because they were candidates for death before they ever came through the door."

There were many red faces in the room by the time he sat down.

ooooo

At the end of my internship, I faced the decision of whether to seek a residency somewhere and specialize, which meant more years of school and more loans, or to become a general practitioner. The choice was clear to me. I wanted to get to work, and I had no burning desire to become a specialist.

I sat for all the exams possible, including the Michigan State, the Canadian Dominion Council, and U.S. National Boards. I received an offer to practice in Ontario, and the chief of staff of St Joseph's in Flint invited me to become his partner.

Polly and I talked it over and decided that neither of us loved cold weather. She'd grown up in Texas, and I had spent many cold nights hitchhiking or slogging my way to and from school on Montreal's snow-choked streets. We decided that California sounded like a good choice.

I discovered that my experience and my boards qualified me to practice in California so I wrote to a placement service in San Francisco. In return, they sent me more than a hundred offers in northern California alone.

The problem was that I was out of money again and had no way to pay for a trip to California. Dr Grady made me an offer I couldn't refuse. He loaned me the money, saying, "I hope you will come back to practice with me. But if you don't, you can pay me back when you're able."

Here was yet another person, another angel with a huge heart, who trusted me. I packed the family and all our belongings in the car and headed off for California. The trip marked the beginning of my true liberation. I had finished my education, and now it was time to take care of people and make a living.

CHAPTER FOURTEEN

FOLLOWING
THE SUN

I had my health back, my family was with me, and the fine western weather reflected my state of optimism. We decided we wanted to live in northern California in a smaller city than Flint but close to a larger city with such cultural amenities as the symphony, opera, and good restaurants.

The hundred or so offers had been organized for me by the placement service giving the location, annual rainfall, average temperature, demographics, local tourist attractions, schools, and expected salary. By the time we had crossed the prairies and the Rockies and were approaching California, Polly and I had narrowed down the candidate cities to twelve.

From a base in Sacramento, we made excursions to the various clinics offering me jobs, turning them down for such reasons as no hospital nearby, too far from San Francisco, too rainy, and so on.

One day we received a telegram that read, "Excellent opening in Fairfield," with no other information. I had no idea where Fairfield was, but on the way back from another interview in Vallejo, we spotted a sign along the road that read, "Fairfield 7 miles." We turned off.

There had been no clue in the terse telegram telling who was looking for a doctor, so we stopped at a car dealership and asked if they had any clues. They sent us across the street to a medical office where the doctor I spoke with just happened to be a McGill graduate, five years ahead of me – Dr Gordon Isaac.

He wasn't looking for a partner, but he thought it had to be a medical group headed by a Dr Ben Stewart which owned a small hospital. Isaac offered to escort us since he was on his way over that direction to see a patient.

We liked the town, and when we got to Stewart's office, I was introduced to him and one of his partners, Dr Frost. They were swamped with patients and asked if could wait until all the patients had been seen. I sat in the waiting room and watched a steady parade of people come and go. Finally, the waiting room was empty and Drs Stewart and Frost invited me into their offices.

The first question they asked was, "When can you start?"

"Tomorrow morning." I said, "But shouldn't we talk about who I am, my training, and my expected salary?"

"We can talk about all that," Stewart said. "We just want to be sure that you can start to work right away."

They offered me $800 a month to start, increasing by $100 every three months.

That sounded a bit convoluted and I needed to have a good steady income right off the bat, so I suggested $1,000 a month for the first year with no raise. They agreed and my future was decided.

ooooo

It took me six years, but I repaid all of those loans that I had nearly killed myself getting while attending McGill.

My career as a general practitioner turned out to be varied. One of the more interesting cases involved a woman whom I admitted to the hospital many times for abdominal pain. Her husband told me to spare no expense treating her. But I could not find the cause of her pain, even after referring her to many specialists in the area, including those at university clinics.

This dragged on for years and it was clear that whatever was causing her pain, at least it wasn't killing her. The diagnosis came unexpectedly during one of the times I admitted her to the hospital for observation. I went to see her the next morning. Neil Armstrong had just stepped on the moon, and she had the TV in her private room tuned to the live coverage.

She was weeping when I walked in. I tried to find out what was troubling her, but she just stared out the window weeping. Suddenly, out of nowhere, an idea hit me like a lightning bolt. Without thinking, I asked, "Do you have a boyfriend?"

She burst into uncontrolled sobbing and I knew I diagnosed her troubles.

She got a grip on herself and we discussed how she was going to resolve her problem. She said she had what she called a boyfriend at the office where she worked, but swore it had been platonic. But now he was pressuring her to go to a hotel to consummate their love.

She and her husband were financially well off, her children were grown and raising families of their own, and she was working just to keep busy. The solution seemed obvious.

"Here's what I'm going to prescribe," I told her. "I'm releasing you this morning. I want you to go to work and put in your resignation, telling them that this is an order from your doctor. Tell them my diagnosis is that the stress of work is causing your abdominal pain." She seemed relieved to have a plan.

She did as I suggested and a few days later, her husband called to say that she was cured. "Doc, she's like a new person. I can't believe after all that it was just the job, and she didn't even need to work."

I never learned what happened with the man she had been flirting with, but she never presented with pain again and I suspect she was feeling trapped between the man, the job, and her husband. Another odd case I encountered early in my career involved a man who was accused of shooting his wife to death before turning the gun on himself. I was making rounds at the hospital when the nurse on duty explained that the man had managed to blow away part of his chest muscle but hadn't damaged any organs. He'd just had surgery and was coming out of the anesthesia. I was to take his vital signs and make sure he was stable.

When I walked into the room, there was a smartly dressed man in a dark suit sitting in a chair next to the bed, holding one of the patient's hands, both of which were handcuffed to the bed rails. A patrolman sat in a chair across the room from the foot of the bed.

The man was moaning a little and when I bent over to have a look at him, he muttered, "Bring me my wife. Where is my wife?"

The well-dressed man leaped to his feet and fixed me with a fierce look. "Did you hear what he said?" he demanded.

"Sure I did. He said, 'Bring me my wife.'"

It was strange, but the guy was coming out of anesthesia and I figured he'd forgotten that he'd killed his wife. But the well-dressed man turned out to be his lawyer, and he made it clear he intended to haul me into court to testify that the patient had asked for his wife. That was going to be part of his defence.

True to his word, the lawyer did subpoena me to testify. The man was convicted, but the judge gave him a lenient sentence because of mitigating circumstances: the shooting was a crime of passion – he had discovered that his wife was cheating on him. Up to that point he had been a leading business figure in the community; he was so remorseful that he had tried to kill himself.

At the other end of the spectrum, there was Olga, a patient I greatly admired. She was an older woman who had suffered from the age of five from tuberculosis of the hip, a devastating illness that causes deformities. Posture becomes tortured, walking painful, and pace snail-like. To walk, she had to use a stupendous effort to heave out her hip just to move her foot a small step forward.

The problem had worsened as she aged. Numerous consultations could come up with no treatment that would restore or rehabilitate her range of movement. This was how I knew her during the many thirty years she was my patient: a person for whom the simplest tasks were Olympian accomplishments.

Yet she rarely complained, carrying herself in every other way as a healthy, pleasant, life-loving person. She enjoyed a good joke, laughed easily and often, and glowed with a mysterious inner beauty.

Near the end of her life, at age sixty-five, she presented her daughter with a pair of red, high-heeled shoes, and instructions for what to do with them upon her death. In her mother's eulogy, her daughter revealed that Olga had wanted to be buried wearing those red shoes. There were audible sobs and few dry eyes among the mourners when her daughter explained, "She wanted to arrive in Heaven ready for dancing."

ooooo

Shakespeare's play *As You Like It* includes a famous soliloquy that, in retrospect, describes my experience as a family-practice physician. The passage begins:

All the world's a stage,
And all the men and women merely players;
They have their exits and their entrances;
And one man in his time plays many parts,
His acts being seven ages.

The rest of the speech describes the seven points on the arc of a human life, from the helplessness of infancy to the helplessness of old age. It is often referred to as the seven ages of man.

In the beginning, my patients tended to be younger people. I delivered a lot of babies but I saw patients with a broad range of issues. In particular, my obstetrical practice provided new patients for some of my pediatric practice.

After fifteen years of delivering babies, spending many sleepless nights and weekends in the delivery room, I abandoned obstetrics. Newfound time for other pursuits was gratifying. I began to see more and more elderly people, more cancer, high blood pressure, heart problems, diabetes, and arthritis.

After another five to ten years, these patients began to show up with more debilitating diseases and I began to build up a large number of nursing home patients. I began to take care of more chronic illnesses, more cancer, more heart failure, and more stroke patients requiring rehabilitation. At one point I had enough patients in the same nursing home that I set aside my day off, Monday, to make rounds there.

This group inevitably led to care of the terminally ill, the hospice patient with only a few months to live. As I completed my third decade in practice, I still had a cross-section of illnesses to treat, but the illnesses of the young were being displaced by those of the elderly.

It had been quite an amazing period of time for technological advances, the thirty years since I graduated from McGill. Diagnostic equipment and treatment techniques had come a long way.

But something else was happening that helped me decide when it was time to hang up my stethoscope. The practice with which I was associated had appointed a "gatekeeper" to review the practices of all the doctors, to make sure we were being as efficient as possible. This was in the late 1980s when HMOs were taking over the business of healthcare and bringing in bean counters to make sure we weren't wasting the investors' money.

Soon after he arrived, the "gatekeeper" called me in to ask why I had ordered a certain test. "It costs us $7.50. Was it really necessary?"

I assured him it was, but his acceptance of my explanation was clearly grudging, as if to say, "Okay, I'll let it go this time. But next time ..."

I'd been practicing medicine for thirty years and it made no sense that my judgment should be subject to scrutiny by a civilian who hadn't examined the patient. The oath I took to heal said nothing about return on investment.

After a few of these gatekeeper inquiries, I realized that medicine had moved on and I should, too. I cut my practice down to three days a week and then cut it out altogether.

But the healing instinct never left me. Polly and I had more time to travel and one day, after visiting Mount Vesuvius in Italy, we returned to our rented car to find next to it a German shepherd, lean and gaunt, with bloody paws, I assumed from walking on the sharp volcanic rocks.

My heart went out to him. He looked abandoned or lost, but definitely without an owner. I remembered all those years ago when the horse and I spent two hours watching each other in a freezing rain. I couldn't do anything for that horse back then, but I could do something for this dog.

I opened the back door and motioned for him to get in. He seemed to understand right away, and slowly pulled himself up into the car and onto the back seat, where he promptly lay down and curled up, looking at me with sad eyes.

There was no food to be had where we were, so we drove down the mountain to a nearby village. I idled slowly down the main street until I spotted a butcher outside his shop, dressing a side of beef. I pulled over and talked to him in Italian as he was cutting off small scraps of meat and tossing them into a pail. I explained that I wanted to pay him for a pail of water to clean the dog's feet, and another for drinking. I also wanted to buy some scraps of meat. He shrugged and agreed.

I coaxed the dog down from the car seat and he plopped on the sidewalk. I could see his paws hurt too much to walk, which was probably why he was starving. I proceeded to wash off the blood and dirt, recalling another unforgettable moment in my life when my mother washed my feet after running in all those races back in high school. As I imagined it was for her, washing the dog's paws was for me a spiritual experience, a manifestation of my faith and an expression of gratitude for my life's many blessings.

The dog drank a lot of water and then bolted down many of the scraps of meat until he finally seemed satiated. I asked the butcher if there was a veterinary hospital nearby. He laughed. "We're lucky we have hospitals for people around here."

So I reached into my wallet and pulled out a large bill. His eyes widened.

"I will give this to you if you make me a solemn promise to feed the dog and care for him until he's able to get on his feet." He gave me a funny look, as though gauging whether I was serious. Then he agreed.

I gave the dog a good scratch behind the ear and said in Italian, "This nice man is going to help you get better. Good luck." I prayed everything would work out for him, just as I had said a prayer for that horse that watched me hitchhiking.

ooooo

Outside of my medical career I had built a second business as a developer of senior apartments and been quite successful at it. Although I was only sixty when I retired from medicine, I stayed busy as a developer, gradually turning over my business interests to my five children so I could have more time for fishing, writing, and reminiscing.

The reminiscing part inevitably took me back to Guelph and a tour of the old neighborhood, which triggered the expected strong emotions of loss and wistfulness. The vacant lots I played in as a child now had houses on them. The street, just two car widths wide, appeared smaller than I remembered. Some of the homes had been renovated, but most looked much as they had when I lived there. The house I grew up in looked just as stark and small as I remembered it. But no one was sitting out on the porches, even though it was summertime. No one was sweeping.

My father's old grocery store had been turned into a residence. Northern Rubber, a large factory across the street from the store, was silent, surrounded by a rusty cyclone fence. Uncle Vincent's shoe repair shop was closed but the building had been ordered preserved by the city as a heritage site. The garage I burned down was never rebuilt, but Borghesi's barn, which also burned that day, had been replaced with a brick structure.

I attended mass at Sacred Heart, recognizing no one in a church where, as a youngster, I knew almost every single person who ever walked through the doors.

The beer store had become the Sikh Special Services Building, and the town had a supermarket for Afghans that sold Halal meats. The telephone book had many Pakistani names in it.

The melting pot of Guelph had new ingredients, but I had no trouble imagining that a young Arab living in post-911 North America experienced some of the same sort of discrimination I did in school as an Italian during World War II. Perhaps sixty years from now, some Afghan-Canadian doctor will write a heartfelt memoir about growing up on Alice Street.

If so, he or she would be continuing a legacy. My brother Pacifico and I sat down in recent years and between us tallied up the list of kids we had known who had turned out all right. There were at least four medical doctors, two veterinary doctors, five attorneys, two engineers, a chemist, a car dealer, many realtors and contractors, two priests, one of whom became bishop of the diocese, three city council members, and countless schoolteachers.

It's not my Alice Street anymore, but it lives on in my memory and now in these pages.